## Praise for **Burnout**

"*Burnout* is the gold standard of self-help books, delivering cutting-edge science with energy, empathy, and wit. The authors know exactly what's going on inside your frazzled brain and body, and exactly what you can do to fix it. . . . Truly life-changing."

—SARAH KNIGHT, *New York Times* bestselling author of *Calm the F\*ck Down*

"In *Burnout*, Emily and Amelia Nagoski deconstruct the stress we experience *as women,* and their compassionate, science-based advice on how to release it made me cry with gratitude and relief. Repeatedly. In public. The book is that revolutionary and its authors that wonderful and wise."

—PEGGY ORENSTEIN, *New York Times* bestselling author of *Girls & Sex: Navigating the Complicated New Landscape*

"Reading *Burnout*, I knew this was not just another self-help book that keeps us trapped by the idea of female inadequacy. It turns our struggle with stress on its head and paves a *meaningful* path to what the authors call 'growing mighty' by bravely dropping in thoroughly contemporary and refreshing truth bombs, like, yeah, the patriarchal system is the issue, and goddamn it's time we play by our own rules!"

—SARAH WILSON, *New York Times* bestselling author of *First, We Make the Beast Beautiful*

"The first sentence of *Burnout* says, 'This is a book for any woman who has felt overwhelmed and exhausted by everything she had to do, and yet still worried she was not doing "enough."' (I raised my hand in bed.) Emily Nagoski [and] her twin sister, Amelia, teamed up to write about how to combat stress, and they have a gift for making the self-help genre not make you want to poke your eyes out."

—Cup of Jo

"*Burnout* excels in its intersectionality. The world is hard for any woman. But certain marginalizations—your skin color, your sexual orientation, your size—can make it even more difficult for certain people. The Nagoskis take these aspects of privilege into account, writing an inclusive narrative that does its best to incorporate as many millennials as possible. . . . A primer on how to stop letting the world dictate how you live and what you think of ourselves, *Burnout* is essential reading."

—*Bustle*

# Burnout

# Burnout

## THE SECRET TO UNLOCKING
## THE STRESS CYCLE

EMILY NAGOSKI, PHD,
AND AMELIA NAGOSKI, DMA

BALLANTINE BOOKS

NEW YORK

2020 Ballantine Books Trade Paperback Edition

Published in the United States by Ballantine Books,
an imprint of Random House, a division of
Penguin Random House LLC, New York.

BALLANTINE and the HOUSE colophon are registered
trademarks of Penguin Random House LLC.

Originally published in hardcover in the United States
by Ballantine Books, an imprint of Random House,
a division of Penguin Random House LLC, in 2019.

LIBRARY OF CONGRESS CATALOGING-IN-PUBLICATION DATA
Names: Nagoski, Emily, author. | Nagoski, Amelia, author.
Title: Burnout : the secret to unlocking the stress cycle /
Emily Nagoski, Ph.D. and Amelia Nagoski, DMA.
Description: First edition. | New York : Ballantine Books, [2019] |
Includes bibliographical references and index.
Identifiers: LCCN 2018051131 (print) | LCCN 2018054198 (ebook) |
ISBN 9781984817075 (Ebook) | ISBN 9781984818324 (trade paperback)
Subjects: LCSH: Stress management. | Women—Health and hygiene. |
BISAC: SELF-HELP / Stress Management. | HEALTH & FITNESS /
Women's Health. | SOCIAL SCIENCE / Women's Studies.
Classification: LCC RA785 (ebook) | LCC RA785 .N35 2019 (print) |
DDC 155.9/042—dc23
LC record available at https://lccn.loc.gov/2018051131

Printed in the United States of America on acid-free paper

randomhousebooks.com

12 14 16 18 19 17 15 13 11

*Book design by Elizabeth A.D. Eno*

For the givers

# TABLE OF CONTENTS

# INTRODUCTION

This is a book for any woman who has felt overwhelmed and exhausted by everything she had to do, and yet still worried she was not doing "enough." Which is every woman we know—including us.

You've heard the usual advice over and over: exercise, green smoothies, self-compassion, coloring books, mindfulness, bubble baths, gratitude. . . . You've probably tried a lot of it. So have we. And sometimes it helps, at least for a while. But then the kids are struggling in school or our partner needs support through a difficulty or a new work project lands in our laps, and we think, *I'll do the self-care thing as soon as I finish this.*

The problem is not that women don't *try.* On the contrary, we're trying all the time, to do and be all the things everyone demands from us. And we will try anything—any green smoothie, any deep-breathing exercise, any coloring book or bath bomb, any retreat or vacation we can shoehorn into our schedules—to be what our work and our family and our world demand. We try to put on our own oxygen mask before assisting others. And then along comes another struggling kid or terrible boss or difficult semester.

The problem is not that we aren't trying. The problem isn't even that we don't know how. The problem is the world has turned "wellness" into yet another goal everyone "should" strive for, but only people with time and money and nannies and yachts and Oprah's phone number can actually achieve.

So this book is different from anything else you'll read about burnout. We'll figure out what wellness can look like in your actual real life, and we'll confront the barriers that stand between you and your own well-being. We'll put those barriers in context, like landmarks on a map, so we can find paths around and over and through them—or sometimes just blow them to smithereens.

With *science*.

## Who We Are and Why We Wrote *Burnout*

Emily is a health educator with a PhD and a *New York Times* bestselling book, *Come as You Are: The Surprising New Science That Will Transform Your Sex Life*. When she was traveling all over talking about that book, readers kept telling her the most life-changing information in the book wasn't the sex science; it was those sections about stress and emotion processing.

When she told her identical twin sister, Amelia, a choral conductor, Amelia blinked like that was obvious. "Of course. Nobody teaches us how to feel our feelings. Hell, I *was* taught. Any conservatory-trained musician learns to feel feelings singing on stages or standing on podiums. But that didn't mean I knew how to do it in the real world. And when I finally learned, it probably saved my life," she said.

"Twice," she added.

And Emily, recalling how it felt to watch her sister crying in a hospital gown, said, "We should write a book about that."

Amelia agreed, saying, "A book about that would've made my life a lot better."

This is that book.

It turned into a lot more than a book about stress. Above all, it became a book about connection. We humans are not built to do big things alone, we are built to work together. That's what we wrote about, and it's how we wrote it.

### IT'S THE *EMOTIONAL EXHAUSTION*

When we told women we were writing a book called *Burnout*, nobody ever asked, "What's burnout?" (Mostly what they said was, "Is it out yet? Can I read it?") We all have an intuitive sense of what "burnout" is; we know how it feels in our bodies and how our emotions crumble in the grip of it. But when it was first coined as a technical term by Herbert Freudenberger in 1975, "burnout" was defined by three components:

1. *emotional exhaustion*—the fatigue that comes from caring too much, for too long;

2. *depersonalization*—the depletion of empathy, caring, and compassion; and

3. *decreased sense of accomplishment*—an unconquerable sense of futility: feeling that nothing you do makes any difference.[1]

And here's an understatement: Burnout is highly prevalent. Twenty to thirty percent of teachers in America have moderately high to high levels of burnout.[2] Similar rates are found among university professors and international humanitarian aid workers.[3] Among medical professionals, burnout can be as high as

52 percent.[4] Nearly all the research on burnout is on professional burnout—specifically "people who help people," like teachers and nurses—but a growing area of research is "parental burnout."[5]

In the forty years since the original formulation, research has found it's the first element in burnout, *emotional exhaustion,* that's most strongly linked to negative impacts on our health, relationships, and work—especially for women.[6]

So what exactly is an "emotion," and how do you exhaust it?

Emotions, at their most basic level, involve the release of neurochemicals in the brain, in response to some stimulus. You see the person you have a crush on across the room, your brain releases a bunch of chemicals, and that triggers a cascade of physiological changes—your heart beats faster, your hormones shift, and your stomach flutters. You take a deep breath and sigh. Your facial expression changes; maybe you blush; even the timbre of your voice becomes warmer. Your thoughts shift to memories of the crush and fantasies about the future, and you suddenly feel an urge to cross the room and say hi. Just about every system in your body responds to the chemical and electrical cascade activated by the sight of the person.

That's emotion. It's automatic and instantaneous. It happens everywhere, and it affects everything. And it's happening all the time—we feel many different emotions simultaneously, even in response to one stimulus. You may feel an urge to approach your crush, but also, simultaneously, feel an urge to turn away and pretend you didn't notice them.

Left to their own devices, emotions—these instantaneous, whole-body reactions to some stimulus—will end on their own. Your attention shifts from your crush to some other topic, and the flush of infatuation eases, until that certain special someone crosses your mind or your path once more. The same goes for the jolt of pain you feel when someone is cruel to you or the flash of disgust when you smell something unpleasant. They just end.

In short, *emotions are tunnels. If you go all the way through them, you get to the light at the end.*

Exhaustion happens when we get *stuck* in an emotion.

We may get stuck simply because we're constantly being exposed to situations that activate emotion—our crush is there, all day, every day, even if only in our thoughts, and so we're trapped in our own longing. Or we return to our stressful job every single day. No wonder "helping professions" are so exhausting—you're confronted with people in need, all day, day after day. No wonder parenting is so exhausting—once you're a parent, you're never not a parent. You're always going through the tunnel.

Sometimes we get stuck because we can't find our way through. The most difficult feelings—rage, grief, despair, helplessness—may be too treacherous to move through alone. We get lost and need someone else, a loving presence, to help us find our way.

And sometimes we get stuck because we're trapped in a place where we are not free to move through the tunnel.

Many of us are trapped in just this way, because of a problem we call "Human Giver Syndrome."

### HUMAN GIVER SYNDROME

In *Down Girl: The Logic of Misogyny,* philosopher Kate Manne describes a system in which one class of people,[7] the "human givers," are expected to offer their time, attention, affection, and bodies willingly, placidly, to the other class of people, the "human beings."[8] The implication in these terms is that human beings have a moral obligation to *be* or *express* their humanity, while human givers have a moral obligation to *give* their humanity to the human beings. Guess which one women are.

In day-to-day life, the dynamic is more complicated and subtle, but let's imagine the cartoon version: The human givers are the "attentive, loving subordinates" to the human beings.[9] The givers' role is to give their whole humanity to the beings, so that the beings can *be* their full humanity. Givers are expected to abdicate any resource or power they may happen to acquire—their jobs, their love, their bodies. Those belong to the beings.

Human givers must, at all times, be *pretty, happy, calm, gener-*

*ous, and attentive to the needs of others,* which means they must never be ugly, angry, upset, ambitious, or attentive to their own needs. Givers are not supposed to need anything. If they dare to ask for or, God forbid, *demand* anything, that's a violation of their role as a giver and they may be punished. And if a giver doesn't obediently and sweetly hand over whatever a being wants, for that, too, the giver may be punished, shamed, or even destroyed.

If we had set out to design a system to induce burnout in half the population, we could not have constructed anything more efficient.

Emotional exhaustion happens when we get stuck in an emotion and can't move through the tunnel. In Human Giver Syndrome, the giver isn't allowed to inconvenience anyone with anything so messy as emotions, so givers are trapped in a situation where they are not free to move through the tunnel. They might even be punished for it.

Your body, with its instinct for self-preservation, knows, on some level, that Human Giver Syndrome is slowly killing you. That's why you keep trying mindfulness and green smoothies and self-care trend after self-care trend. But that instinct for self-preservation is battling a syndrome that insists that self-preservation is *selfish,* so your efforts to care for yourself might actually make things worse, activating even more punishment from the world or from yourself, because how dare you?

Human Giver Syndrome is our disease.

The book you're reading is our prescription.

## How the Book Is Organized

We've divided *Burnout* into three parts. Part I is "What You Take with You."

In the Star Wars movie *Episode V: The Empire Strikes Back,*

Luke Skywalker sees an evil cave. Looking toward the entrance in dread, he asks his teacher Yoda, "What's in there?"

Yoda answers, "Only what you take with you."

This beginning section of the book explains three internal resources that we carry with us as we take our heroine's journey: the stress response cycle, "the Monitor" (the brain mechanism that controls the emotion of frustration), and meaning in life. Meaning is often misunderstood as "the thing we'll find at the end of the tunnel," but it's not. It's why we go through the tunnel, regardless of what we find on the other end. (Spoiler alert: meaning is good for us.)

Which brings us to Part II. We call it "The Real Enemy."

That's a reference to *The Hunger Games,* in which young Katniss Everdeen is forced into a "game" organized by the dystopian sci-fi government, in which she has to kill other children.

Her mentor says to her, "Remember who the real enemy is." It's not the people the government wants her to kill, and who are trying to kill her. The real enemy is the government that set this whole system up in the first place.

Can you guess what the enemy is in this book?

[Cue ominous music] The Patriarchy. Ugh.

Most self-help books for women leave this chapter out and instead discuss only the things readers can control, but that's like teaching someone the best winning strategy of a game without mentioning that *the game is rigged*. Fortunately, when we understand how the game is rigged, we can start playing by our own rules.

And then Part III—the thrilling conclusion—is the science of winning the war against these "real enemies." It turns out there are concrete, specific things we can do each and every day, to grow mighty and conquer the enemy.

We call this part "Wax On, Wax Off."

In the original *Karate Kid* movie, Mr. Miyagi teaches Danny LaRusso karate by having the kid wax his car.

"Wax on," says Mr. Miyagi, rotating his palm clockwise. "Wax off," he says, rotating his other palm counterclockwise, and he adds, "Don't forget to breathe." He also has Danny sand the deck, stain the fence, and paint the house.

Why the repetitive, mundane tasks?

Because in the mundane tasks live the protective gestures that help us grow strong enough to defend ourselves and the people we love, and to make peace with our enemies.

"Wax on, wax off" is *what makes you stronger*: connection, rest, and self-compassion.

Throughout the book, you'll follow the stories of two women: Julie, an overwhelmed public school teacher whose body will revolt against her, forcing her to pay attention to it; and Sophie, an engineer who will decide she is not here for the patriarchy. These women are composites: In the same way a movie is made of thousands of still images, edited together to tell a story, they are composed of fragments of dozens of real-life women. We're using this technique partly to protect the identities of the real women and partly because this larger narrative arc more effectively explains the science than stand-alone vignettes can. The research doesn't come close to addressing every woman's experience, but we hope that these stories will give you that sense of how each individual's experience is unique and yet, at the same time, universal.

And each chapter ends with a "tl;dr" list. *Tl;dr* is the Internet abbreviation for "too long; didn't read." If you write a five-hundred-word post on Facebook or a multiparagraph comment on Instagram, someone may well reply, "tl;dr." Our tl;dr lists contain the ideas you can share with your best friend when she calls you in tears, the facts you can use to disprove myths when they come up in conversation, and the thoughts we hope come to you when your racing mind keeps you awake at night.

## A CAVEAT OR TWO ABOUT SCIENCE

In this book, we use science as a tool to help women live better lives. We've turned to diverse domains of science, including affective neuroscience, psychophysiology, positive psychology, ethology, game theory, computational biology, and many others. So a few words of caution about science.

Science is the best idea humanity has ever had. It's a systematic way of exploring the nature of reality, of testing and proving or disproving ideas. But it's important to remember that science is ultimately a specialized way of being *wrong*. That is, every scientist tries to be (a) slightly less wrong than the scientists who came before them, by proving that something we thought was true actually isn't, and (b) wrong in a way that can be tested and proven, which results in the next scientist being slightly less wrong. Research is the ongoing process of learning new things that show us a little more of what's true, which inevitably reveals how wrong we used to be, and it is never "finished." So whenever you read a headline like "New Study Shows . . ." or "Latest Research Finds . . . ," read with skepticism. One study does not equal proof of anything. In *Burnout,* we've aimed to use ideas that have been established over multiple decades and reinforced by multiple approaches. Still, science doesn't offer perfect truth, only the best available truth. Science, in a sense, is not an exact science.

A second caveat: Social science is generally done by measuring lots of people and assessing the average measurement of all those people, because people *vary*. Just because something is true about a group of people—like, American women are, on average, five feet four inches tall—doesn't mean it's true about any specific individual within that group. So if you meet an American woman who isn't five foot four, there's nothing wrong with her, she's just different from the average. And there's nothing wrong with the science, either; it's true that women are, on average, five foot four—but that tells us nothing in particular about any specific woman we may meet. So if you read some science in this book that describes "women" but doesn't describe you, that doesn't mean the science is wrong and it doesn't mean there's something wrong with you. People vary, and they change. Science is too blunt an instrument to capture every woman's situation.

A third caveat: Science is often expensive, and who pays for it can influence the outcome and whether or not the results are published. As enthusiastic as we are about evidence-based practices, it's important to remember where that evidence comes from and why we might not see contrary evidence.[10]

Science has a fourth specific limitation worth mentioning in a book about women: When a research article says it studied "women," it almost always means it studied people who were born in a body that made all the grown-ups around them say, "It's a girl!" and then that person was raised as a girl and grew into an adult who felt comfortable in the psychological identity and social role of "woman." There are plenty of people who identify as women for whom at least one of those things is not true, and there are plenty of people who *don't* identify as women, for whom one or more of those things is true. In this book, when we use the word "woman," we mostly mean "people who identify as women," but it's important to remember that when we describe the science, we're limited to the women who were identified at birth and raised as women, because that's mostly who has been studied. (Sorry.)

So. We try to be as science-based as we can be, but we're aware of its limits.

That's where the art comes in.

As science fiction author Cassandra Clare writes, "Fiction is truth, even if it is not fact." This is what storytelling is for—and in fact research has found that people understand science better when it's communicated through storytelling! So side by side with the neuroscience and computational biology, we'll talk about Disney princesses, sci-fi dystopias, pop music, and more, because story goes where science can't.

## THE OWL AND THE CHEESE

Here's a real study that real scientists really conducted:[11]

Research participants were given some mazes—just lines on paper—and instructed that their goal was to get the cartoon mouse from one side of the maze to the other. In one version of the maze, a cartoon owl loomed over the page, hunting the mouse. In another version, a morsel of cheese awaited the mouse at its destination.

Which group completed the maze faster, the ones who were moving toward the cheese, or the ones who were fleeing from the owl?

The cheese group. Participants completed more mazes, more quickly, when their imaginations were propelled toward a reward even as mild as cartoon cheese, than when running away from an uncomfortable state even as subtle as the threat of a cartoon owl.

It makes perfect sense when you think about it. If you're moving toward a specific, desired goal, your attention and efforts are focused on that single outcome. But if you're moving away from a threat, it hardly matters where you end up, as long as it's somewhere safe from the threat.

The moral of the story is: We thrive when we have a positive goal to move *toward,* not just a negative state we're trying to move away from. If we hate where we are, our first instinct often is to run aimlessly away from the owl of our present circumstances, which may lead us somewhere not much better than where we started. We need something positive to move toward. We need the cheese.

The "cheese" of *Burnout* isn't just feeling less overwhelmed and exhausted, or no longer worrying whether you're doing "enough." The cheese is *growing mighty,* feeling strong enough to cope with all the owls and mazes and anything else the world throws at you.

Our promise to you is this: Wherever you are in your life, whether you're struggling in a pit of despair and searching for a way out, or you're doing great and want tools to grow mightier, you will find something important in these pages. We'll show you science that proves you're normal and you're not alone. We'll offer evidence-based tools to use when you're struggling and that you can share with people you love when they're struggling. We'll surprise you with science that contradicts the "common-sense" knowledge you've spent your whole life believing. And we'll inspire and empower you to create positive change in your own life and the lives of those you love.

Writing this book did all of these things for us—showed us we're normal and we're not alone, taught us important skills to use when we're struggling, and surprised us and empowered us. It has already changed our lives, and we think it will change yours, too.

## PART I

## What You Take with You

# 1

## COMPLETE THE CYCLE

*"I've decided to start selling drugs so I can quit my job."*

*This is how Amelia's friend Julie recently answered the question "How are you?" the Saturday before the new school year started. She was kidding, of course . . . except she wasn't. She's a middle school teacher. Her burnout had reached an intensity where merely the anticipation of the start of the first semester had activated a level of dread that left her reaching for the box of Chardonnay by 2 P.M.*

*Nobody likes to think of their kids' middle school teacher as burned out, embittered, and day-drinking, but she's not alone. Burnout—with its cynicism, sense of helplessness, and, above all, emotional exhaustion—is startlingly ubiquitous.*

*"I saw that story about the teacher who showed up on the first day of school drunk with no pants, and I thought, 'There but for the grace of God go I,'" Julie told Amelia, from the bottom of her first glass.*

*"Dread is anxiety on steroids," Amelia said, remembering her own days teaching middle school music, "and the anxiety comes from the accumulation, day after day, of stress that never ends."*

*"Yes," Julie declared, filling her glass again.*

*"The thing about teaching is, you can't ever get rid of the causes of the stress," Amelia said. "And I don't mean the kids."*

*"Right?" Julie agreed. "The kids are why I'm there. It's the administration and the paperwork and that crap."*

*"And you can't get rid of those kinds of stressors," Amelia said, "but you can get rid of the stress itself, when you know how to complete the stress response cycle."*

*"Yes," Julie said again, emphatically. Then she said, "What do you mean, 'complete the cycle'?"*

This chapter is the answer to Julie's question, and it might be the most important idea in the book: Dealing with your *stress* is a separate process from dealing with the things that cause your stress. To deal with your *stress*, you have to *complete the cycle.*

## "Stress"

Let's start by differentiating our *stress* from our *stressors.*

*Stressors* are what activate the stress response in your body. They can be anything you see, hear, smell, touch, taste, or imagine could do you harm. There are external stressors: work, money, family, time, cultural norms and expectations, experiences of discrimination, and so on. And there are less tangible, internal stressors: self-criticism, body image, identity, memories, and The Future. In different ways and to different degrees, all of these things may be interpreted by your body as potential *threats*.

*Stress* is the neurological and physiological shift that happens in your body when you encounter one of these threats. It's an evolutionarily adaptive response that helps us cope with things like, say, being chased by a lion or charged by a hippo.[1] When your brain notices the lion (or hippo), it activates a generic "stress response," a cascade of neurological and hormonal activity that initiates physiological changes to help you survive: epinephrine acts instantly to push blood into your muscles, glucocorticoids keep you going, and endorphins help you ignore how uncomfortable all of this is. Your heart beats faster, so your blood pumps harder, so your blood pressure increases and you breathe more quickly (measures of cardiovascular functioning are a common way researchers study stress).[2] Your muscles tense; your sensitivity to pain diminishes; your attention is alert and vigilant, focusing on short-term, here-and-now thinking; your senses are heightened; your memory shifts to channel its functioning to the narrow band of experience and knowledge most immediately relevant to this stressor. Plus, to maximize your body's efficiency in this state, your other organ systems get deprioritized: Your digestion slows down and your immune functioning shifts (measures of immune function are another common way researchers study stress).[3] Ditto growth and tissue repair, as well as reproductive functioning. Your *entire body and mind* change in response to the perceived threat.

And so here comes the lion. You are flooded with stress response. What do you do?

You *run*.

You see, this complex, multisystem response has one primary goal: to move oxygen and fuel into your muscles, in anticipation of the need to escape. Any process not relevant to that task is postponed. As Robert Sapolsky puts it, "For us vertebrates, the core of the stress-response is built around the fact that your muscles are going to work like crazy."[4]

So you run.

And then?

Well, then there are only two possible outcomes: either you get eaten by the lion (or trampled by the hippo—in either case, none of the rest of this matters) or else you escape! You survive! You run back to your village, the lion chasing you all the while, and you shout for help! Everyone comes out and helps you slaughter the lion—you're saved! Yay! You love your friends and family! You're grateful to be alive! The sun seems to shine more brightly as you relax into the certain knowledge that your body is a safe place to be. Together, the village cooks a lot of the lion and shares a communal feast, and then you all bury the parts you can't use, in an honoring ceremony. Hand in hand with the people you love, you take a deep, relaxing breath and give thanks to the lion for its sacrifice.

Stress response cycle complete, and we all live happily ever after.

## Just Because You've Dealt with the *Stressor* Doesn't Mean You've Dealt with the *Stress Itself*

Our stress response is beautifully fitted to the environment where it evolved. The behavior that dealt with a lion was the behavior that completed the stress response cycle. And that makes it easy to assume that it's the elimination of the lion—the cause of the stress—that completed the cycle.

But no.

Suppose you were running away from the lion, when it's struck by lightning! You turn and see the dead lion, but do you suddenly feel peaceful and relaxed? No. You stop, puzzled, heart pounding, eyes darting in search of the threat. Your body still wants to run or fight or hide in a cave and cry. The threat may have been dealt with by an act of God, but you're left still needing to do something to let your body know you're safe. The stress response cycle needs to complete, and just eliminating the stressor isn't enough to do that. So maybe you run back to your village and breathlessly tell your tribe what happened, and you all jump up and down and cheer and thank God for the lightning bolt.

Or a modern example: Suppose the lion charges—it's coming right for you! Adrenaline and cortisol and glycogen, oh my! And so, thinking quickly, you grab your rifle and shoot the lion, to save your own life. Bang. The lion drops dead.

Now what? The threat is gone, but again your body is still in full action mode, because you haven't done anything your body recognizes as a cue that you are safe. Your body is stuck in the middle of the stress response. Just telling yourself, "You're safe now; calm down," doesn't help. Even seeing the dead lion isn't enough. You have to do something that signals to your body that you are safe, or else you'll stay in that state, with neurochemicals and hormones degrading but never shifting into relaxation. Your digestive system, immune system, cardiovascular system, musculoskeletal system, and reproductive system never get the signal that they're safe.

But wait, there's more:

Suppose the stressor is not a lion, but some jerk at work. This jerk will never be a threat to our lives, he's just a pain in the ass. He says some jerky thing at a meeting, and you get a similar flood of adrenaline and cortisol and glycogen, oh my.[5] But you have to sit there in that meeting and be "nice." "Socially appropriate." It would only escalate the situation if you vaulted across the table and scratched his eyes out, as your physiology is telling you to do. Instead, you have a quiet, socially appropriate, highly functional meeting with his supervisor, in which you recruit the supervisor's support in intervening the next time the jerk says another jerky thing.

Congratulations!

But addressing the cause of the stress doesn't mean you've addressed the stress itself. Your body is soaked in stress juice, just waiting for some cue that you are now safe from the potential threat and can relax into celebration.

And it happens day after day . . . after day.

Let's think about what this does to just one system, the cardiovascular: Chronically activated stress response means chronically increased blood pressure, which is like constantly turning a firehose on in your blood vessels, when those vessels were designed by evolution to handle only a gently flowing stream. The increased wear and tear on your blood vessels leads to increased risk for heart disease. That's how chronic stress leads to life-threatening illness.

And this happens, remember, in every organ system in your body. Digestion. Immune functioning. Hormones. We are not built to live in that state. If we get stuck there, the physiological response intended to save us can instead slowly kill us.

This is the upside-down world we live in: in most situations in the modern, post-industrial West, the stress itself will kill you faster than the stressor will—*unless* you do something to complete the stress response cycle. While you're managing the day's stressors, your body is managing the day's stress, and it is absolutely essential to your well-being—the way sleeping and eating are absolutely essential—that you give your body the resources it needs to complete the stress response cycles that have been activated.

Before we talk about how to do that, let's talk about why we aren't already doing it.

## Why We Get Stuck

There are lots of reasons why the cycle might not complete. These are the three we see most often:

*1. Chronic Stressor* → *Chronic Stress.* Sometimes your brain activates a stress response, you do the thing it says, and it doesn't change the situation:

"Run!" it says, when you're confronted by a terrifying project—speaking in front of a group of your peers, say, or writing a giant report or interviewing for a job.

So you "run," in your twenty-first-century way: when you get home that day, you put on Beyoncé and dance it out for half an hour.

"We escaped the lion!" your brain says, breathless and grinning. "Self high five!" And you're rewarded with all kinds of feel-good brain chemicals.

And then tomorrow . . . the terrifying project is still there.

"Run!" your brain says again.

And the cycle begins again.

We get stuck in the stress response, because we're stuck in a stress-activating situation. That's not always bad—it's only bad when the stress outpaces our capacity to process it. Which, alas, is a lot of the time, because . . .

*2. Social Appropriateness.* Sometimes the brain activates a stress response and you can't do the thing it's trying to tell you to do:

"Run!" it says, pumping out adrenaline for you.

"I can't!" you say. "I'm in the middle of an exam!"

Or, "Punch that asshole in the face!" it says, dumping glucocorticoids into your bloodstream.

"I can't!" you say. "He's my client!"

So you sit politely and smile benignly and do your best, while your body stews in stress juice, waiting for you to do something.

And sometimes the world tells you it's *wrong* to feel that stress—wrong for so many reasons, in so many ways. It's not nice; it's weak; it's impolite.

Many of us were raised to be "good girls," to be "nice." Fear and anger and other uncomfortable emotions can cause distress in the people around you, so it's not nice to feel those things in front of other people. We smile and ignore our feelings, because our feelings matter less than the other person's.

And also it's *weak* to feel those feelings, our culture has taught us. You're a smart, strong woman, so when you're walking down the street and a guy shouts, "Nice tits!" you tell yourself to ignore it. You tell yourself you're not in danger, it's irrational to feel angry or afraid, and anyway, that guy isn't worth it, he doesn't matter.

Meanwhile, your brain shouts, "Gross!" and makes you walk faster.

"What?" the guy who isn't worth it calls after you. "Can't you take a compliment?"

"Just ignore it," you tell yourself, swallowing the adrenaline. "You're too strong to be affected by this."

But it's not just that it's not nice, and it's not just that it's weak, it's that it's *impolite,* we're taught. When your cousin posts a misogynistic comment on Facebook, you could YELL AT HIM FOR REPEATING NONSENSE THAT IS NOT MERELY FACTUALLY INCORRECT BUT ALSO MORALLY WRONG OMFG I CAN'T BELIEVE I EVEN STILL HAVE TO SAY THESE THINGS. Then he—and probably several other people—will respond that you might have a point, but he can't listen to you when you're so shrill. So angry. You need to make your point more *politely* if you want to be taken seriously.

Be nice, be strong, be polite. No feelings for you.

3. *It's Safer.* Is there a strategy for dealing with, say, street harassment, that deals with both the situation and the stress caused by the situation? Sure. Turn around and slap that guy in the face. But then what? Will he suddenly realize that street harassment is bad and thus stop doing it? Probably not. More likely, the situation will escalate and he'll hit you, in which case it just got way more dangerous. Sometimes walking away is the win. Smiling and being nice, ignoring it and telling yourself it doesn't matter— these are survival strategies. Use them with pride. Just don't for-

get that these survival strategies do not deal with the stress itself. They postpone your body's need to complete the cycle; they don't replace it.

So many ways to deny, ignore, or suppress your stress response! For all these reasons and more, most of us are walking around with decades of incomplete stress response cycles simmering away in our chemistry, just waiting for a chance to complete.

And then there's freeze.

## Freeze

We've been talking about the stress response in the familiar terms of "fight or flight." When you feel threatened, the brain does a split-second assessment to determine which response is more likely to result in your survival. *Flight* happens when your brain notices a threat and decides that you're more likely to survive by trying to escape. That's what happens when you run from a lion. *Fight* happens when your brain decides you're more likely to survive the threat by trying to conquer it. From a biological point of view, fight and flight are essentially the same thing. Flight is fear—avoidance—whereas fight is anger—approach—but they're both the "GO!" stress response of the sympathetic nervous system. They tell you to *do something*.

Freeze is special. Freeze happens when the brain assesses the threat and decides you're too slow to run and too small to fight, and so your best hope for survival is to "play dead" until the threat goes away or someone comes along to help you. Freeze is your last-ditch stress response, reserved for threats that the brain perceives as life-threatening, when fight or flight don't stand a chance. In the middle of the gas pedal of stress response, your brain slams on the brakes—the parasympathetic nervous system swamping the sympathetic—and you shut down.

Imagine you're a gazelle running away from a lion. You're midflight, full of adrenaline—but you feel the lion's teeth chomp into your hip. What do you do? You can't run anymore—the lion has hold of you. You can't fight—the lion is much stronger. So your nervous system slams on the brakes. You collapse and play dead. That's freeze.

You don't have to know about freeze in order for your brain to choose it, but if you don't know that freeze exists, you may think about a circumstance where you were unsafe and wonder why you didn't kick and scream, why you didn't fight or run—why, in fact, you felt as if you *couldn't* scream or kick or run. The reason is that you really couldn't. Your brain was trying to keep you alive in the face of a threat that seemed unsurvivable, so it slammed on the brakes in a last-ditch attempt to do that.

And you know what? It worked. Here you are. Alive and reading a book about stress. Hello! We're really glad you're here. We're grateful to your brain for keeping you alive.

---

### "THE FEELS"

Our culture gives us a lot of ways to describe what it feels like when your brain chooses the "Go!" stress responses. When your brain chooses fight, you may feel *irritated, annoyed, frustrated, angry, irate,* or *enraged.* When it chooses flight, we have words to describe that feeling: *unsure, worried, anxious, scared, frightened,* or *terrified.* But what are the words that describe the emotion of "freeze"? Words that might feel right: *Shut down. Numb. Immobilized. Disconnected. Petrified.* The very word *sympathetic* means "with emotion," while *parasympathetic*—the system that controls freeze—means "*beyond* emotion." You may feel disengaged from the world, sluggish, like you don't care or nothing matters. You feel... outside.

If we don't have a good word to describe the experience of freeze, we really don't have a good word to describe what comes next:

After a gazelle freezes in response to a lion attack, the lion, feeling smug, wanders off to get her cubs so they can feed on the gazelle. And that's when the magic happens: Once the threat is gone, the brake gradually eases off, and the gazelle begins to shake and shudder. All the adrenaline and cortisol built up in her bloodstream get purged through this process, the same way running to safety purges those chemicals.

It happens in all mammals. One woman, when she learned about freeze, told us, "So that's what happened to a cat I accidentally hit with my car—she was just lying there and I was terrified she was dead; I felt terrible. Then she started twitching and shaking and I thought she was having a seizure, until it was like she woke up . . . and then ran away."

It happens to humans, too. People have told us, "That happened to my friend, when she was coming out from under anesthesia after surgery."

And, "My kid went through that in the emergency room."

And, "When I was coming to terms with a trauma I experienced, sometimes my body would go into this state where I felt out of control, and it scared me because I felt out of control during the trauma itself. Now I know it was actually my body taking care of me; it was part of my healing."

We don't have words for the experience of having the brake come off—the shaking, shuddering, muscle-stretching, involuntary response that is often accompanied by waves of rage, panic, and shame. If you don't know what it is, it can feel scary. You might try to fight it or control it. That's why it's so important that we give it a name: We call it "the Feels," and it's nothing to fear. It's a normal, healthy part of completing the cycle, a physiological reaction that will end on its own, usually lasting just a few minutes. Feels usually happen in extreme cases where the stress response cycle is interrupted suddenly and not allowed to complete. It's part of the healing process following a traumatic event or long-term, intense stress.

Trust your body. The sensations may bring awareness of their origins, or they may not; doesn't matter. Awareness and insight are not required in order for the Feels to move through you and out of you. Crying for no apparent reason? Great! Just notice any apparently causeless emotions or sensations or trembling and say, "Ah. There's some Feels."

## The Most Efficient Way to Complete the Cycle

When you're being chased by a lion, what do you do?

You run.

When you're stressed out by the bureaucracy and hassle of living in the twenty-first century, what do you do?

You run.

Or swim.

Or dance around your living room, singing along to Beyoncé, or sweat it out in a Zumba class, or do literally anything that moves your body enough to get you breathing deeply.

For how long?

Between twenty and sixty minutes a day does it for most folks.

And it should be most days—after all, you experience stress most days, so you should complete the stress response cycle most days, too. But even just standing up from your chair, taking a deep breath, and tensing all your muscles for twenty seconds, then shaking it out with a big exhale, is an excellent start.

Remember, your body has no idea what "filing your taxes" or "resolving an interpersonal conflict through rational problem-solving" means. It knows, though, what jumping up and down means. Speak its language—and its language is *body* language.

You know how everyone says exercise is good for you? That it helps with stress and improves your health and mood and intelligence and basically you should definitely get some?[6] This is why. Physical activity is what tells your brain you have successfully survived the threat and now your body is a safe place to live. *Physical activity is the single most efficient strategy for completing the stress response cycle.*

## Other Ways to Complete the Cycle

Physical activity—literally any movement of your body—is your first line of attack in the battle against burnout. But it's not the only thing that works to complete the stress response cycle—far from it! Here are six other evidence-based strategies:

*Breathing.* Deep, slow breaths downregulate the stress response—especially when the exhalation is long and slow and goes all the way to the end of the breath, so that your belly contracts. Breathing is most effective when your stress isn't that high, or when you just need to siphon off the very worst of the stress so that you can get through a difficult situation, after which you'll do something more hardcore. Also, if you're living with the aftermath of trauma, simply breathing deeply is the gentlest way to begin unlocking from the trauma, which makes it a great place to start. A simple, practical exercise is to breathe in to a slow count of five, hold that breath for five, then exhale for a slow count of ten, and pause for another count of five. Do that three times—just one minute and fifteen seconds of breathing—and see how you feel.

*Positive Social Interaction.* Casual but friendly social interaction is the first external sign that the world is a safe place. Most of us expect we'll be happier if, say, our seatmate on a train leaves us alone, in mutual silence; turns out, people experience greater well-being if they've had a polite, casual chat with their seatmate.[7] People with more acquaintances are happier.[8] Just go buy a cup of coffee and say "Nice day" to the barista. Compliment the lunch lady's earrings. Reassure your brain that the world is a safe, sane place, and not all people suck. It helps!

*Laughter.* Laughing together—and even just reminiscing about the times we've laughed together—increases relationship satisfaction.[9] We don't mean social or "posed" laughter, we mean belly laughs—deep, impolite, helpless laughter. When we laugh, says neuroscientist Sophie Scott, we use an "ancient evolutionary system that mammals have evolved to make and maintain social bonds and regulate emotions."[10]

*Affection.* When friendly chitchat with colleagues doesn't cut it, when you're too stressed out for laughter, deeper connection with a loving presence is called for. Most often, this comes from some loving and beloved person who likes, respects, and trusts you, whom you like, respect, and trust. It doesn't have to be physical affection, though physical affection is great; a warm hug, in a safe and trusting context, can do as much to help your body feel like it has escaped a threat as jogging a couple of miles, and it's a heck of a lot less sweaty.

One example of affection is the "six-second kiss" advice from relationship researcher John Gottman. Every day, he suggests, kiss your partner for six seconds. That's one six-second kiss, mind you, not six one-second kisses. Six seconds is, if you think about it, a potentially awkwardly long kiss. But there's a reason for it: Six seconds is too long to kiss someone you resent or dislike, and it's far too long to kiss someone with whom you feel unsafe.

Kissing for six seconds requires that you stop and deliberately notice that you like this person, that you trust them, and that you feel affection for them. By noticing those things, the kiss tells your body that you are safe with your tribe.

Another example: Hug someone you love and trust for twenty full seconds, while both of you are standing over your own centers of balance. Most of the time when we hug people, it's a quick, lean-in type hug, or it might be a longer hug where you each lean on each other, so that if one person lets go, the other person would fall over. Instead, support your own weight, as your partner does the same, and put your arms around each other. Hold on. The research suggests a twenty-second hug can change your hormones, lower your blood pressure and heart rate, and improve mood, all of which are reflected in the post-hug increase in the social-bonding hormone oxytocin.[11]

Like a long, mindful kiss, a twenty-second hug can teach your body that you are safe; you have escaped the lion and arrived home, safe and sound, to the people you love.

Of course, it doesn't have to be precisely twenty seconds. What matters is that you feel the shift of the cycle completing. Therapist Suzanne Iasenza describes it as "hugging until relaxed."

Happily, our capacity to complete the cycle with affection doesn't stop with other human beings. Just petting a cat for a few minutes can lower your blood pressure, and pet owners often describe their attachment to their pets as more supportive than their human relationships.[12] No wonder people who walk their dogs get more exercise and feel better than people who don't— they're getting exercise and affection at the same time.[13] And for people whose experiences have taught them that no one is trustworthy, therapies with horses, dogs, and other animals can open a door to the power of connection.

Our capacity to complete the cycle with affection doesn't even stop at connection with mundane life on Earth. Often when researchers examine the role of spirituality in a person's well-being, they talk about "meaning in life"—which is so important we've got a whole chapter on it (chapter 3)—or about the social support provided by fellow members of a religious community. But a spiritual connection is also about feeling safe, loved, and supported by a higher power. In short, it's about feeling connected to an invisible yet intensely tangible tribe.[14]

*A Big Ol' Cry.* Anyone who says "Crying doesn't solve anything" doesn't know the difference between dealing with the stress and dealing with the situation that causes the stress. Have you had the experience of just barely making it inside before you slam the door behind you and burst into tears for ten minutes? Then you wipe your nose, sigh a big sigh, and feel relieved from the weight of whatever made you cry? You may not have changed the situation that caused the stress, but you completed the cycle.

Have a favorite tearjerker movie that makes you cry every time? You know exactly when to grab the tissues and sniff, "I love this part!" Going through that emotion with the characters allows your body to go through it, too. The story guides you through the complete emotional cycle.

*Creative Expression.* Engaging in creative activities today leads to more energy, excitement, and enthusiasm tomorrow.[15]

Why? How? Like sports, the arts—including painting, sculpture, music, theater, and storytelling in all forms—create a context that tolerates, even encourages, big emotions. In the first flush of romantic love, for example, all those songs on the radio suddenly make sense! And those songs keep us company even when our friends are rolling their eyes and sick of hearing about how in love we are. And when we are heartbroken, there's a playlist to lead us through the tunnel of our grief and keep us company as we move through it, to a place of peace. In this way, literary, visual, and performing arts of all kinds give us the chance to celebrate and move through big emotions. It's like a cultural loophole in a society that tells us to be "nice" and not make waves. Take advantage of the loophole.

Writers and painters and creators of all kinds have said the same thing one Nashville songwriter told us: "Looking back at my very first songs, it's completely obvious that I was dealing with my past, and trying to process my trauma history into something meaningful. At the time, I was completely in denial— I didn't even know I *had* pain. But writing songs helped me feel what my mind had hidden from me. My songs were a safe place to put what I couldn't deal with otherwise."[16]

*Sophie is an engineer and a* Star Trek *geek and a lot of other things, but she is not an athlete. In high school, people saw a six-foot-one black girl and told her she should play basketball, and she told them where they could put their basketball. She hates exercise. She will not exercise. In fact, if she ever tries to exercise, after a few days she inevitably comes down with something or is injured, or a project comes up that means she doesn't have time anymore. She can't exercise. Can't. Hates it, can't do it, won't do it.*

*So when Emily visited her office to lead a lunchtime seminar about stress and said, "Exercise is good for you," Sophie approached her afterward.*

*"You don't understand, Emily. It's boring and painful and every time I do it, something goes wrong. I can't, I won't, I don't want to, just no. No. I'm not going to exercise. I don't care how good it is for my stress."*

*Not everyone is a natural exerciser. But the research is so unambiguous that exercise is good for you that, as a health educator, Emily has searched for ways to support people who can't exercise or hate exercise or just don't exercise, for whatever reason. When she looked at the research, to her astonishment, most of the conclusions said things like "Join a team sport" or "Make it a hobby, not just exercise!" In other words, the advice said, "Find a way to enjoy exercise!" Which is good advice, but not for someone with chronic pain or illness, injury or disability, or someone like Sophie who will. Not. Exercise.*

*But then Emily found a remarkable branch of research on body-based therapies, whose results she applies to folks like Sophie. Here's what Emily suggested.*

*"Okay, so just lie in bed—"*

*"My favorite sport," Sophie said.*

*"Then just progressively tense and release every muscle in your body, starting with your feet and ending with your face. Tense them hard, hard, hard, for a ssslllooowww count of ten. Make sure you spend extra time tensing the places where you carry your stress."*

*"Shoulders," Sophie said instantly.*

*"Super! And while you do that, you visualize, really clearly and viscerally, what it feels like to beat the living daylights out of whatever stressor you've encountered."*

*"Okay," Sophie said with some enthusiasm.*

*"Imagine it really clearly, though—that matters a lot. You should notice your body responding, like your heart beating faster and your fists clenching, until you reach a satisfying sense of—"*

*"Victory," Sophie said. "I got this."*

*She did. And strange things started to happen. Sometimes, when she was doing the muscle-tension activity, she felt inexplicable waves of frustration and anger. Occasionally, she'd cry. Sometimes her body would seem to take over and shake and shudder in strange ways, as if she were possessed.*

*She emailed Emily about it.*

*"Totally normal," Emily assured her. "That's your baggage unpacking itself. All those incomplete stress response cycles that have built up inside you are finally releasing. Trust your body."*

There are so many ways to complete the cycle, it's not possible to catalogue all of them here. Physical activity, affection, laughter, creative expression, and even just breathing have something in common as strategies, though: you have to *do something*.

One thing we know for sure doesn't work: just telling yourself that everything is okay now. Completing the cycle isn't an intellectual decision; it's a physiological shift. Just as you don't tell your heart to continue beating or your digestion to continue churning, the cycle doesn't complete by deliberate choice. You give your body what it needs, and allow it to do what it does, in the time that it requires.

## How Do You Know You've Completed the Cycle?

It's like knowing when you're full after a meal, or like knowing when you've had an orgasm. Your body tells you, and it's easier for some people to recognize than others. You might experience it as a shift in mood or mental state or physical tension, as you breathe more deeply and your thoughts relax.

For some people, it's as obvious as knowing that they're breathing. That's how it is for Emily. Long before she knew about the science, she knew that when she felt stressed and tense and terrible, she could go for a run or for a bike ride and at the end of it she would feel better. Even on the days when she looked at her shoes and thought, *Ugh, I just don't want to,* she knew that on the other side of those shoes and that run or that ride was peace. Once, she even cried at the top of a hill in southeastern Pennsylvanian farm country, breathing hard and marveling at the smell of cows and the glow of sunlight on the pavement, as the gears of her bike whirred under her. She has always been able to feel it intuitively, the shift inside her body.

How does it feel?

It's a gear shift—a slip of the chain to a smaller gear, and all of a sudden the wheels are spinning more freely. It's a relaxation in her muscles and a deepening of her breath.

The more regularly she exercises, the more easily she gets

there. If she has let the stress accumulate inside her for days or weeks, one workout won't get her all the way there. She'll feel better at the end of a run, but not *done*. If you've spent a long time accumulating incomplete stress response cycles inside your body, you may have this experience, too. When you begin practicing strategies to complete the cycle, you'll feel only some relief at first, not necessarily the full relaxation of completion. That's okay, too.

For others—like Amelia—recognizing when the cycle completes is not so intuitive. She was in her therapist's office, feeling anxious, the first time she noticed it happening. The therapist asked her to describe what her anxiety felt like, and Amelia waxed poetic for about four minutes, talking about the tension in her shoulders and the heat in her neck and the quivering in her hair follicles, then stopped to breathe.

"And how do you feel now?" the therapist asked.

"Um. I . . . I don't know. I can't find it anymore. I think it's just . . . gone?"

"Yeah. That's how it works. If anxiety starts, it ends."

"It *just ends*?"

"Yeah. If you let it, it just ends."

We asked a group of therapists how they could tell they had completed the cycle. One therapist talked not about herself, but about her young daughter. When her daughter came to her in distress, she would hold her, as a mother does, and watch her face as she cried. Gradually, the taut muscles in the little girl's face and body would soften, and she would give a great big shuddering sigh, and then she'd be able to talk about what had happened to cause the distress. The big sigh was the signal that her little body had made the shift.[17]

Don't worry if you're not sure you can recognize when you've "completed" the cycle. Especially if you've spent a lot of years—like, your whole life, maybe—holding on to your worry or anger, you've probably got a whole lot of accumulated stress response cycles spinning their engines, waiting for their turn, so it's going to take a while before you get through the backlog. All you need to do is recognize that you feel *incrementally better* than you felt before you started. You can notice that something in your body has changed, shifted in the direction of peace.

"If I was at an eight on the stress scale when I started, I'm at a four now," you can say. And that's pretty great.

## The Practical Advice

The "how to" here is very simple:

First, find what works. It would be convenient if we could just tell you which strategy will work best for you, but you'll probably find that different strategies work better on different days, and sometimes the strategy that works best isn't practical day to day, so you need a backup strategy. You can probably already think of a few things that feel right, but experiment, then schedule that stuff into your day. Put it in your calendar. Thirty minutes of anything that works for you: exercise, meditation, creative expression, affection, etc. Because you experience stress every day, you have to build completing the cycle into every day. Make it a priority, like your life depends on it. Because it does.

Remember, Emily intuitively understood completing the cycle from early adolescence, while Amelia, genetically identical and raised in the same household, didn't even begin to understand until after years of therapy, two hospitalizations for stress-induced inflammation, formal meditation training, and explicit instruction from her health educator sister. So we know everybody's different. But with practice, you'll begin to notice what different stress levels feel like in your body, and you'll get a sense of which days require more or less time or intensity to complete the cycle.

For a lot of people, the most difficult thing about "completing the cycle" is that it almost always requires that they stop dealing with whatever caused the stress, step away from that situation, and turn instead toward their own body and emotions.

By this point in the chapter, you know that dealing with the stressor and dealing with the stress are two different processes, and you have to do both. You have to, or else your stress will gradually erode your well-being until your body and mind break down.

## Signs You Need to Deal with the Stress, Even If It Means Ignoring the Stressor

Your brain and body exhibit predictable signs when your stress level is elevated, and these serve as reliable cues that indicate you need to deal with the stress itself before you can be effective in dealing with the stressor.

1. *You notice yourself doing the same, apparently pointless thing over and over again, or engaging in self-destructive behaviors.* When your brain gets stuck, it may start stuttering or repeating itself, like a broken record, or like a breathless eight-year-old trying to get her mother's attention by saying "Guess what? Guess what? Guess what?" You might notice yourself checking things, picking at things, thinking obsessive thoughts, or fiddling with your own body in a routinized kind of way. These are signs that the stress has overwhelmed your brain's ability to cope rationally with the stressor.

2. *"Chandeliering."* This is Brené Brown's term for the sudden, overwhelming burst of pain so intense you can no longer contain it, and you jump as high as the chandelier. It's out of proportion to what's happening in the here and now, but it's not out of proportion to the suffering you're holding inside. And it has to go somewhere. So it erupts. That eruption is a sign you're past your threshold and need to deal with the stress before you can deal with the stressor.

3. *You turn into a bunny hiding under a hedge.* Imagine a rab-

bit being chased by a fox, and she runs under a bush to hide. How long does she stay there?

Until the fox is gone, right?

When your brain is stuck in the middle of the cycle, it may lose the ability to recognize that the fox has gone, so you just stay under that bush—that is, you come home from work and watch cat videos while eating ice cream directly from the container, using potato chips for a spoon, or stay in bed all weekend, hiding from your life. If you're hiding from your life, you're past your threshold. You aren't dealing with either the stress or the stressor. Deal with the stress so you can be well enough to deal with the stressor.

4. *Your body feels out of whack.* Maybe you're sick all the time: you have chronic pain, injuries that just won't heal, or infections that keep coming back. Because stress is not "just stress," but a biological event that really happens inside your body, it can cause biological problems that really happen inside your body but can't always be explained with obvious diagnoses. Chronic illness and injury can be caused or exacerbated by chronic activation of the stress response.

*Amelia told Julie the story of how the science of completing the cycle saved her life (twice).*

*"It was when I was in grad school. I was trying to do something that mattered a lot to me, while simultaneously battling this totally dysfunctional administration—"*

*"Oh my God, that's so familiar," Julie said.*

*"—and the stress built up inside me in layers that got denser and denser until they finally crushed me. Halfway through the program, I was hospitalized with abdominal pain and a white blood cell count that was through the roof. They couldn't find a cause; they sent me home and told me to 'relax.'"*

*"Whatever that means," Julie said.*

*"I didn't know either! I just knew I had to do something. So I started noticing all the external stressors that activated my stress and recognizing how little control over them I had, so I could start letting go of those things. I feel sure it helped save my life. But it wasn't enough. A year later, I was back in the hospital and they took out my appendix—the pressing layers of stress inside me had finally destroyed an organ."*

*"Stress can do that?"*

*"Heck yes,"* Amelia said. *"So my sister visited me in the hospital. She brought me a book about inflammation."*

*"Your sister gave you a book while you were in the hospital?"*

*"And a balloon that sang 'Don't Worry Be Happy,' which also helped,"* Amelia said. *"But this book explained how health conditions like repeated infections, chronic pain, and asthma—all of which I had—are exacerbated or even caused by stress. By unprocessed emotion. I got home and read this book, and I just started crying, even though I was thinking,* That's nonsense. *It sounded like hippy-dippy bullshit. But, dude, I was in so much pain all the time, and it was getting worse as I got older. So I called Emily sobbing, like, 'This book says emotions exist in the body. Is that true?'"*

*"Okay, wow,"* Julie said. *"Even I knew that."*

*"That's what I'm saying. If I can learn to deal with the stress itself, learn to complete the cycle, you can, too. Anyone can.*

*"Anyway, I asked Emily what I was supposed to do with all this emotion and pain and crap in my body, and she drove an hour and a half to my house, to bring me a book of relaxation meditations."*

*"Because of course Emily would give you a book,"* Julie said.

*"Exactly. So I started using these meditations on the treadmill and elliptical machine, paying attention to physical sensations and recognizing for the first time that certain stray thoughts corresponded with specific bodily discomforts. It was wild. It was mind-blowing. And it worked. I'm healthier—and saner and happier—than I was in my twenties, because I realized my emotions and my thoughts and my body are all connected to one another. Now I'm the one who nags her to exercise and cry and write fiction when she needs to."*

*"Because those are the ways she completes the cycle," Julie observed. "Okay." She twisted her wineglass between her fingers, thinking.*

*Julie made a plan. She started the school year with two new strategies: She would begin sifting controllable stressors from uncontrollable stressors, and she would practice completing the cycle. She set aside half an hour a day, six days a week, for exercise or pure play with her daughter, Diana.*

*It helped . . . but a few months later she hit a serious obstacle. And that's the subject of the next chapter.*

The good news is that stress is not the problem. The problem is that the strategies that deal with stressors have almost no relationship to the strategies that deal with the physiological reactions our bodies have to those stressors. To be "well" is not to live in a state of perpetual safety and calm, but to move fluidly from a state of adversity, risk, adventure, or excitement, back to safety and calm, and out again. Stress is not bad for you; *being stuck* is bad for you. Wellness happens when your body is a place of safety for you, even when your body is not necessarily in a safe place. You can be well, even during the times when you don't feel good.

———

Here's the ultimate moral of the story:

> Wellness is not a state of being, but a state of action.

Our job in this chapter has been to teach you how to deal with the *stress* so that you can be well enough to face another day of stressors.

But of course, that still leaves you with a life full of goals, obstacles, unmet obligations, not-yet-fulfilled hopes, and other sources of stress, both big and small, both enjoyable and painful.

So let's talk about those goals, and the brain mechanism that keeps track of them.

## tl;dr:

- Just because you've dealt with a stressor, that doesn't mean you've dealt with the stress itself. And you have to deal with the stress—"complete the cycle"—or it will slowly kill you.

- Physical activity is the single most efficient strategy for completing the cycle—even if it's just jumping up and down or a good old cry.

- Affection—a six-second kiss, a twenty-second hug, six minutes of snuggling after sex, helpless laughter—are social strategies that complete the cycle, along with creative self-expression—writing, drawing, singing, whatever gives you a safe place to move through the emotional cycle of stress.

- "Wellness" is the freedom to move fluidly through the cycles of being human. Wellness is thus not a state of being; it is a state of action.

## 2

## #PERSIST

*Sophie, the non-exerciser, is an engineer, but she's also a black woman, so she rarely gets to be just an engineer. She has to be an engineer and a social justice educator, teaching the oblivious white guys who surround her about the experience of being a woman of color in science and technology—not because she wants to; all she ever wanted to do is science. But since she is so often the only person of color and the only woman in the room, they all look to her to explain, ya know, why she's the only person of color or woman in the room.*

*One day as we were sitting around a table at an end-of-semester breakfast with her and a bunch of other women, Sophie told us a story about the ways she was being taken for granted on a "diversity" committee she'd been assigned to.*

*"Is it . . . racism?" Emily said hesitantly, a white lady afraid to hurt anyone's feelings. "Is it because you're a woman?"*

*"It's just the usual nonsense," Sophie said. "I'm used to all that."*

*Amelia, not hesitant, said, "What is wrong with them? Isn't it obvious that putting people of color in charge of helping white people learn how not to be racist is just more white supremacy? White people are the ones with the problem; we should be doing the work, not putting more labor demands on black and brown people."*

*Sophie grinned at her omelet and said, "Actually . . . I've been thinking, if they're going to ask me to do all this, I can turn it into a way to get paid. Codify a package of talks and workshops. Take the Sophie Show on the road. I get requests all the time."*

*"Can we talk about the science of how smart that idea is?" Emily said, excited and impressed. "There's so much research about how to turn our frustrations into assets."*

*"Can we talk about the science?" Sophie echoed. "Let's always talk about the science!"*

*This chapter is that science.*

Chapter 1 was about dealing with the stress itself. Chapter 2 is about managing the stressors. It's about knowing how to persist when you're past the edge of your capabilities, and it's about knowing when to quit. Specifically, it's about what we call "the Monitor," the brain mechanism that manages the gap between where we are and where we are going. Exactly what this looks like is different for everyone, but it impacts every domain of life, from parenthood to career success to friendships to body image. And for women, the gap quickly becomes a chasm.

In this chapter, we'll explain how the Monitor works, and why it sometimes breaks down. Then we'll talk about how to implement evidence-based strategies for every frustration and every failure, from traffic jams to tenure.

## Allow Us to Introduce . . . the Monitor

Technically, it's called the "discrepancy-reducing/-increasing feedback loop" and "criterion velocity," but people fall asleep immediately when we say that, so we just call it the Monitor. It is the brain mechanism that decides whether to keep trying . . . or to give up.

The Monitor knows (1) what your goal is; (2) how much effort you're investing in that goal; and (3) how much progress you're making. It keeps a running tally of your effort-to-progress ratio, and it has a strong opinion about what that ratio should be. There are so many ways a plan can go wrong, some of which you can control and some of which you can't, all of which will frustrate your Monitor.[1]

For example, imagine you're working toward a simple goal: driving to the mall. And you know it usually takes about, say, twenty minutes. If you're getting all green lights and you're zipping right along, that feels nice, right? You're making progress more quickly and easily than your Monitor expects, and that feels great. Less effort, more progress: satisfied Monitor.

But suppose you get stuck at a traffic light because someone isn't paying attention. You feel a little annoyed and frustrated, and maybe you try to get around that jerk before the next light. But once you've hit one red light, you end up stuck at every traffic light, and with each stop, your frustration burns a little hotter. It's already been twenty minutes, and you're only halfway to the mall. "Annoyed and frustrated" escalates to "pissed off." Then you get on the highway, and there's an accident! While ambulances and police come and go, you sit there, parked on the highway for forty minutes, fuming and boiling and swearing never to go to the mall ever again. High investment, little progress: ragey Monitor.

But then! If you sit there long enough, an enormous emotional shift happens inside you. Your Monitor switches its assessment of your goal from "attainable" to "unattainable," and it pushes you off an emotional cliff, into a *pit of despair*. Lost in helplessness, your brain abandons hope and you sit in your car sobbing, because all you want to do now is go home, and there's nothing you can do but sit there and wait.

In an almost painfully funny video posted in January 2017, the satirical news website The Onion reported that "an increasing number of women are leaving the workplace to pursue lying facedown on the floor full-time. A Department of Labor report says lying motionless in utter resignation on nights and weekends is just no longer enough for most women." That's the pit of despair: resignation and helplessness.

The tremendous power of understanding the Monitor is that once we're aware of how it works, we can influence our own brain's functioning, with strategies for dealing with both the controllable and the uncontrollable stressors.

## Dealing with Stressors You Can Control: Planful Problem-Solving

The Monitor keeps track of your effort and your progress. When a lot of effort fails to produce a satisfying amount of progress, we can change the *kind* of effort we're investing. For example, the frustration of being stuck in traffic can be minimized with a GPS giving you a new route to go around the traffic. All you need to do is make sure you've got the GPS handy. This strategy is called planful problem-solving.

If you carry a purse laden with the complete contents of a drugstore, you already know about planful problem-solving. If you write lists, keep calendars, or follow a budget, you know what planful problem-solving entails. It does what it says on the label: you analyze the problem, you make a plan based on your analysis, and then you execute the plan. The good news is that women are socialized to planfully solve problems. The bad news is that every problem calls for a specific kind of planning.

For example, if we're talking about, say, managing cancer treatment while working full-time and raising your kids and being a partner to someone, there are a lot of calendars involved, and information about medication side effects and how they're managed, and strategies for making sure everyone gets fed and does their homework and gets where they need to go each day. Or if you're trying to find a job, there's the routine of looking for postings, sending résumés, attending networking events, prepping for interviews, and so on. There are pragmatic steps to manage the controllable factors, and controlling what you can control makes the rest of it more bearable.

The least intuitive part of planful problem-solving is managing the stress caused by the problems and the solving. As we learned in chapter 1, what works to manage your stressor will rarely help you manage the stress, so remember to build *completing the cycle* into your plan.

Which brings us to the effective way to deal with *un*controllable stressors.

## Dealing with Stressors You *Can't* Control: Positive Reappraisal

So imagine that you're stuck in traffic and your GPS is busted. For this situation, the strategy we turn to is "positive reappraisal."[2]

Positive reappraisal involves recognizing that sitting in traffic is *worth* it. It means deciding that the effort, the discomfort, the frustration, the unanticipated obstacles, and even the repeated failure have value—not just because they are steps toward a worthwhile goal, but because you reframe difficulties as opportunities for growth and learning.[3]

Some people naturally notice what's valuable in difficult situations. These natural optimists expect good things to happen and automatically believe that bad things, if they happen, are temporary, isolated events that will have no lasting impact. If that's you, congratulations! Optimism is associated with all kinds of positive outcomes related to mental health, physical health, and relationships.[4] You probably don't need any more persuasion or instruction on positive reappraisal. You just keep on keeping on—see the silver lining of every cloud and the rainbows of every storm. Do you.

Pessimists, by contrast, don't always expect good outcomes and may view bad things, if they happen, as symptomatic of larger-scale problems that could have lasting impact. Amelia is the most pessimistic person we know—we've measured it objectively, with survey instruments used to assess pessimism and optimism—and, moreover, she's a conductor whose professional training teaches her that she can and should be responsible for *everything*. So she did not buy this "positive reappraisal" thing. It sounded to her like a video a friend of ours shared on Facebook titled "Eight Things Happy People Do Differently." It included such helpful if idiomatically capitalized gems as "EXPRESS GRATITUDE—never let the things you WANT make you forget about the things you HAVE" and "CULTIVATE OPTIMISM. Stay positive. When it rains, look for Rainbows. When it's dark, look for Stars."

That is not what "positive reappraisal" means; it's not as simple as "look on the bright side" or "find the silver lining" or "enjoy the journey." Nor is it about not feeling frustrated by the persistent gap between what is and what could or should be. Nor does it mean sticking your fingers in your ears and going, "La la la, nothing is wrong, everything is fine!" With positive reappraisal, you can acknowledge when things are difficult, and you recognize that the difficulty is worth it—it is, in fact, an *opportunity*.

So Emily presented a couple of decades' worth of peer-reviewed science to Amelia, who had no problem with the first two steps: first, acknowledge when things are difficult; then, acknowledge that the difficulty is worth it. Pessimists assume everything is hard and will require work, so that's easy. The hard part is acknowledging that those difficulties are actually opportunities.

But positive reappraisal works because it's genuinely true that difficulties are opportunities! When something feels uncomfortable, you're probably doing something that creates more and better progress than if it were easy. Just a handful of examples: Students whose assigned reading is typed in an ugly, difficult-to-read font remember more of what they read in the short term and score higher on exams in the longer term than those whose materials are more legible.[5] A noticeable, annoying buzz of background noise can increase a person's creativity.[6] Groups that are more heterogeneous generate more innovation and better solutions to problems, even though those groups feel less confident about their solution and find the process more difficult.[7] And, most straightforwardly, people who challenge their bodies with regular exercise develop stronger bones, muscles, and cardiovascular systems—strength is the body's response to doing something effortful.

In fact, there is a distinct downside to effort that is too effortless: When a task feels easy, we feel more confident about our ability to perform that task even though we are actually *more likely to fail*. Novices who are thoroughly incompetent rate themselves as very confident in their ability to do a thing they've just learned to do. By contrast, genuine experts know how difficult their work is, so they are realistic about their competence and thus rate their confidence in their own abilities as moderate, even as their performance is, of course, expert-level.

The reduced stress of positive reappraisal is not an illusion.

Struggle can increase creativity and learning, strengthen your capacity to cope with greater difficulties in the future, and empower you to continue working toward goals that matter to you. Reappraisal even changes our brain functioning: The dorsolateral prefrontal cortex activates, which damps the ventromedial prefrontal cortex, which damps the amygdala, which reduces the stress response.[8] Not every kind of stressor is explicitly beneficial, of course. Knowing you're being compared with other people, for example, is quite likely to reduce creativity.[9] But often, the uncomfortable or frustrating process is more successful. As the researchers put it, you can "convert affective pains into cognitive gains."[10]

## Change the Expectancy: Redefine Winning

Planful problem-solving and positive reappraisal are evidence-based ways to change the effort you invest as you move toward a goal. They'll reduce your frustration by keeping you motivated and moving forward. But suppose you do all that, and it works . . . except . . . it's much more difficult or much . . . slower . . . than . . .

you . . .

expected.

Even as you're succeeding, you grow frustrated because your progress is not meeting your Monitor's expectation about how effortful the task should be. In this case, you need to change your Monitor's expectancies about how difficult it will be or how long it will take.

Expectancies are the plan. "Twenty minutes to the mall" is an expectancy. "Four years to finish my degree" is another. So is "married with a kid by the time I'm thirty." When you're frustrated by the slow or interrupted progress toward your goal, and planful problem-solving and positive reappraisal don't help with the frustration, you need to redefine winning. Here's how:

Say your goal is to climb Mount Everest. If you start marching up the mountain expecting that you're going to zip smoothly to the peak, as soon as it gets difficult your Monitor will start to freak out. You might give up. You might start to wonder if there's something wrong with you—after all, somebody told you it was supposed to be easy, and it turns out it's hard, so it's not the mountain that's the problem, it's *you*!

But if you begin the climb knowing ahead of time that it's going to be the most difficult thing you've ever done, then when it begins to get difficult, your Monitor will recognize that without getting frustrated. It's just a difficult goal, so it's normal that you're struggling.

If you're trying to do something where you will inevitably fail and be rejected repeatedly before you achieve your goal—like, if you're recording music or you're an actor or you sell insurance or you're trying to raise a teenager to be a reasonable adult—then you will need a nonstandard relationship with winning, focusing on incremental goals.

Amelia tested this strategy one summer, at a choral recording session.

If you were to imagine a recording session, you might visualize a group of musicians jamming together for hours, or maybe a singer in gigantic headphones, singing her heart out into a microphone, and the musicians leave hours later, filled with the joy of artistic expression.

Maybe that's what it's like sometimes. But most of the time, a musical recording session is more like being stuck in heavy traffic on your way home from work. It's stop-and-go, when all you want to do is get home.

In a recording session, the goal is *perfection,* and humans are not perfect, so it's six measures (maybe fifteen seconds of music) over and over, with a guy behind a window saying, "Great singing, choir; let's do one more," in between.

After twenty minutes of singing the same six measures of music over and over . . . you start to get bored. After forty minutes, the music no longer has feeling. And then the guy behind the window says, "Lovely singing, choir. It sounds a little dry. Can we make the color more specific this take?" And you want to rip your hair out, because no, we can't make the color more specific, because all the neurotransmitters associated with emotional (and therefore timbral) specificity were burned up fifteen minutes ago when measure two was out of tune. So, no.

But you have to. It's a recording session, and the goal is *perfection*—every take, every snippet, every moment. Six to eight hours of artistic and vocal perfection is the goal.

"So we have two choices," Amelia said to a choir of forty professional singers. "We can stuff the frustration down deep where it will cause us to explode at someone else at a later date or otherwise adversely affect our art and our health . . . or we can redefine winning.

"The goal, with each take," Amelia proposed, "is to fill Andrew with joy."

Andrew was their guy behind the window, the recording engineer—and not just any recording engineer. Andrew was the Grammy-winning recording engineer who had worked with some of the most prestigious performers of the twenty-first century. It didn't hurt that he was also a cutie patootie—blond, British, bashful. Everyone in the choir was pretty giddy to be working with him.

Forty singers smiled at the possibility of filling Andrew with joy, and the energy in the room shifted.

"It's better already, isn't it?" Amelia observed.

It was.

On the third day of trying to fill Andrew with joy, when it was getting pretty tough to stay focused but they still had another track to lay down, a soprano asked Andrew, "Andrew, are you filled with joy?"

Andrew paused in moving a microphone cable, considered for a moment, and nodded. He said, "Yeah. I really am."

Redefining winning made the recording session far less agonizing. But better still, a year later, when the group met again, several singers approached Amelia privately to tell her, "That Monitor thing? That's changed, like, my whole life."

You'll find a worksheet at the end of the chapter to help you brainstorm incremental goals that will keep your Monitor satisfied, but the super-short guidelines are: *soon, certain, positive, concrete, specific,* and *personal.*[11] *Soon:* Your goal should be achievable without requiring patience. *Certain:* Your goal should be within your control. *Positive:* It should be something that feels good, not just something that avoids suffering. *Concrete:* Measurable. You can ask Andrew, "Are you filled with joy?" and he can say yes or no. *Specific:* Not general, like "fill people with joy," but specific: Fill *Andrew* with joy. *Personal:* Tailor your goal. If you don't care about Andrew's state of mind, forget Andrew. Who is your Andrew? Maybe you're your own Andrew.

Redefining winning in terms of incremental goals is not the same as giving yourself rewards for making progress—such rewards are counterintuitively ineffective and may even be detrimental.[12] When you redefine winning, you set goals that are *achievements in themselves*—and success is its own reward.

## Change the Expectancy: Redefine Failing

For goals that are abstract, impossible, or otherwise intangible, you can reduce frustration by establishing a nonstandard relationship with winning. But sometimes you're aiming for a clearly defined, concrete goal that can't be redefined. For these, you will need a nonstandard relationship with *failing*. You may do all the things you're supposed to do, without getting where you're trying to go, only to end up somewhere else pretty amazing. Or, as Douglas Adams's character Dirk Gently puts it, "I rarely end up where I was intending to go, but often I end up somewhere that I needed to be." Widen your focus to see the inadvertent benefits you stumble across along the way. This sort of reframing makes failing almost (*almost*) impossible, since it acknowledges that there's more to success than winning.

And we don't just mean the "We played our best!" spirit of your six-year-old's soccer team. There are endless examples of people not achieving their specific goal but achieving something important, something world-changing, along their path to failure. Post-it notes were invented when a chemist tried and failed to make a strong glue; it turned out his very weak glue had a very popular use. The pacemaker was invented when Wilson Greatbatch was trying to create an instrument to measure heart rate, and he built his prototype wrong. Hillary Clinton's failure to win the White House set the stage for record-breaking numbers of women to enter and win political contests and other leadership positions in the United States. Post-its and pacemakers and a tidal wave of women entering American politics were world-changing outcomes of someone's failure to accomplish something else.

It's the most demanding form of positive reappraisal, and none of this takes away the pain of failure and loss. Part of recovering from a loss is turning toward your grief with kindness and compassion, as well as completing the cycle of stress brought on by failure. But another part is recognizing failing's unintended positive outcomes.

### HOW NOT TO MANAGE YOUR MONITOR

Planful problem-solving and positive reappraisal are the adaptive coping strategies, meaning they generally work and they carry minimal risk of unwanted consequences. There are other coping strategies that don't necessarily help, and some strategies that are actively destructive. These maladaptive strategies include things like self-defeating confrontation, suppressing your stress, and avoidance. We often turn to such strategies when we feel out of control in a stressful situation and are desperately trying to regain control.

An example of self-defeating confrontation is, "I stood my ground and fought!" Standing our ground is important in principle and can be effective when we're not overwhelmed, but not when we're stressed and out of control. When you're still fighting even while you're overwhelmed, it's less a valiant struggle and more that you have your back to the wall and are surrounded on all sides. Ask for help instead.

Suppressing is, "I didn't let it get to me." If something matters, it should get to you! It should activate a stress response cycle. Denying that you experience the stress prevents you from dealing with the stress—and we know from chapter 1 what happens if you do that. If you notice yourself acting as though you're fine when you're deeply distressed, again: ask for help.

Avoidance has a couple different flavors. There's "I waited for a miracle to happen," which abdicates personal responsibility for creating change, and there's "I ate until I couldn't feel my feelings," which numbs you out. These can both be useful stop-gap measures when the stress, worry, frustration, rage, or despair are overwhelming. Sometimes we need to numb out with Netflix and a pint of Häggen-Dazs. Once, Emily was teaching about "completing the cycle" and the importance of actually feeling your feelings and one person asked, "Is this true if you're, like, caring for a terminally ill parent? Is it bad to just shut everything out sometimes and spend all day watching *Pride and Prejudice*?"

Heck no. Sometimes you need to close the door

on the world and allow yourself to feel comfortable and safe—as long as it's not the only thing you're doing. Think of it as a short-term survival strategy. You also need a plan and a sense of what value there is in the struggle.

Perhaps the most reliably maladaptive response to distress is "rumination." Like a cow chewing its cud, we regurgitate our suffering over and over, gnawing on it to extract every last bit of pain. If you find your thoughts and feelings go back again and again to your suffering, ask for help.

*"This is why people quit self-care," Julie said to Amelia, opening a bakery box to reveal a gooey chocolate cake. She cut a big slice. "When you paint the dingiest wall in a room, it just makes the other walls look dingier. You said, 'Process your stress, which is separate from processing the stressor.' Well, I did that, and it helped, and now I'm thinking about getting a divorce, and it's basically because of you. Dig in!" She offered a slab of cake on a plate.*

*"What the huh?" Amelia said, accepting the slab.*

*"The huh" was that Julie had spent a month learning to recognize the stressors in her life, and then completing her stress response cycles. That was all it took for her to notice that one of her chronic stressors was her husband, Jeremy.*

*"I started noticing how much work I was putting into managing his feelings," she said, "how much additional stress I had because of his stress. Then last week it was Diana's fall recital, and I told Jeremy, 'It's time to go,' and he groaned, 'All those kids and that terrible music,' and I tried to make him feel better, you know? It's not*

*like this is my first choice for spending three hours of my life, but this is what we do. So I said, 'This is a special moment. We get to see our daughter on stage,' trying to help him see the bright side. And you know what he said? He said, 'You can make me go but you can't make me like it.' Make him go! Make him like it! Recitals are parenting! Why am I having to 'make' him parent?! And why am I having to make him feel better? Nobody makes me feel better, I have to do that myself! I have to find things to enjoy about things that are not enjoyable. I have to find a way not to complain about things I don't like or want in my life. So that night, we got into a fight about it, and he said, 'Well, if you don't want to do it, don't do it. Don't try to make me feel good. Don't try to look on the bright side. Complain if you want to!'*

"So that's what I did. Usually, my first instinct is to just do something myself because he never does it—the dishes, the laundry, wiping the kitchen counters—and instead I complained. And you'll never guess what happened. A week later, he said, 'What's wrong with you? All you do is complain and criticize! You're so negative!' I'm so negative! Can you believe that? I said, 'You told me to complain when I wanted to complain. You said don't try to manage your feelings. And if I'm not managing your feelings then I'm telling you that just running the dishwasher does not count as cleaning the kitchen.'

"And then he says—brace yourself for this—he says, 'You know, if you want something done your way, you have to do it yourself.'"

"Hence considering divorce," Amelia said.

"Except sometimes it's great. It's amazing," Julie said. She stopped for more cake, washing it down with dark beer, then she went on, "You know how slot machines are designed to hook you? Like, most of the time, you're just shoving good money after bad, but every now and then it *pays out just enough to make you feel like you should keep going? That's my marriage," Julie said. "So I quit. I don't know what I quit, I don't know for how long, but I quit. I quit everything but chocolate cake."*

*It's normal for change to be difficult. Sometimes it gets worse before it gets better. Sometimes a solution to one problem creates another. Sometimes there's not enough organization and positive attitude in the world to save a marriage. Sometimes—as Julie would eventually find— what it takes to save a marriage is saving yourself.*

## When to Give Up

The Monitor has a pivot point, where it switches its assessment of your goal from "attainable" to "unattainable." You may find yourself oscillating between pushing onward and giving up, between frustrated rage—"This goal *is* attainable, and screw these jerks in my way!"—and helpless despair—"I can't do it, I give up, everything is terrible!"

It's easier to manage emotions effectively when we can name them.[13] We couldn't find a name for this emotion, even though every person we know has experienced it. So we gave it a name: "Foop."

You can call it whatever feels right for you, but we like this silly word. We experience it at difficult jobs, as in "I hate this place, I hate these people, I'm going to quit! But no, I'm trapped here, I need the money, I have to wait until I have a new job lined up, I'm never getting out of this hole!" You're stuck in Foop Town. It happens in school, as in "I'm going to finish this semester and nothing and no one can stop me, no matter how much crap they throw at me! Ugh, I can't do it, I give up, I'm a failure!" Foop-o-rama. It happens in difficult relationships, as in "I'm sure I can save this relationship, I just need to try harder!

But no, it's hopeless, they'll never change, I'm not good enough at feelings to help them be a better person, but ugh, it's not my job to change them! But ugh, I should change *me*." Über-foop.

So how do you know when it's time to stop the planful problem-solving, drop the positive reappraisal, and just . . . quit?

Science has an answer for when to walk away—sort of. It's framed in terms of an "explore/exploit problem," as in "Should I explore new terrain, or should I exploit the terrain I'm in?" Animals in the wild are good at it.

Imagine a little bird or a squirrel searching for seeds and nuts in a patch of forest. At a certain point, she'll spend more and more time searching, with less and less success, as she discovers and hoards most of the available food in that patch. Her Monitor is well tuned to the environment and automatically triggers a decision to move on to the next patch. It's not a rational, cognitive decision; her instincts are connected to the world, reading the environment, and they signal her to move on, taking into account the cost of the change, including traveling to a new patch, risk of predation, and so on.[14]

If you want to try using this principle rationally, all you have to do is write four lists:

What are the benefits of continuing?

What are the benefits of stopping?

What are the costs of continuing?

What are the costs of stopping?

And then you look at those four lists and make a decision based on your estimates of maximizing benefit and minimizing cost. Remember to consider both the long-term and the short-term costs and benefits. And if you decide to continue, remember to include completing the cycle in your plan.

**DECISION GRID**

*Should I stay or quit:* _____

_____ *(e.g., my job, my relationship, my diet, my place of worship, my substance use, my habit of overcommitting . . .)*

| STAYING THE SAME | QUITTING |
|---|---|
| BENEFITS—IMMEDIATE: | BENEFITS—IMMEDIATE: |
| BENEFITS—LONGER-TERM | BENEFITS—LONGER-TERM |
| COSTS—IMMEDIATE: | COSTS—IMMEDIATE: |
| COSTS—LONGER-TERM | COSTS—LONGER-TERM |

But a lot of the time, knowing when to give up comes to us not from rational, explicit cost-benefit analysis; it comes to us the same way it comes to the bird and the squirrel—in a quiet intuition that is outside rationality. We simply hear the voice inside us saying, "You've done all you can here. It's time to move on."

Humans—especially women—have an extraordinary capacity to ignore this voice. We live in a culture that values "self-control," "grit," and persistence. Many of us are taught to see a shift in goals as "weakness" and "failure," where another culture would see courage, strength, and openness to new possibilities. We have been taught that letting go of a goal is the same as failing. We share stories of people overcoming the odds to achieve remarkable things in the face of great resistance, which is inspiring. But these stories too often imply that we are the controllers of our destinies—as if we control the amount of nuts and seeds in a particular patch of forest. If we "fail" to achieve a goal, it's because there is something wrong with us. We didn't fight hard enough. We didn't "believe."

Our tendency to cling to the broken thing we have rather than let it go and reach for something new isn't just a result of social learning. The stress (fear, anxiety, etc.) underlying the belief *changes our decision-making*, so that the more stressed we feel about change, the less likely we are to do it. Say a squirrel hears a noise in the leaves somewhere close by, so she stops for a moment, listens . . . hears nothing else. But she's vigilant now. Her stress response is activated. And she stays foraging in her current patch, because there's more risk in trying a new patch, what with that potential hidden predator rustling the leaves. It doesn't matter how many more nuts and seeds are in the next patch if there's also a hawk there that will eat her.

And the resource abundance of the environment you're in changes how you decide to quit or stay. In a resource-rich environment, people actually quit and move on to the next opportunity sooner, because the risk of the move is lower. It's easier to change jobs when you've got four offers. It's easier to leave a bad relationship when you can go straight to a loving relationship with someone else.

For so many reasons, quitting is hard, and we can't tell you what the right decision is. But knowing the factors that shape our reluctance to give up, we can say this: If you're feeling not just frustrated and challenged, but helpless, isolated, and trapped, like you want to hide in a cave, or like you'd rather put your hand in a toilet full of tadpoles than spend one more day doing the thing, you should definitely quit whatever it is.

## #ShePersisted

Massachusetts senator Elizabeth Warren made news when, as she was attempting to speak in the Senate, she was silenced by Senate Majority Leader Mitch McConnell. Senator Warren's goal, when McConnell stopped her, was to read a letter from Coretta Scott King about the racist judicial record of then-Senator Jeff Sessions. McConnell said, in what would become a notorious comment, "She was warned. She was given an explanation. Nevertheless, she persisted."

Senators Tom Udall, Sherrod Brown, Bernie Sanders, and Jeff Merkley subsequently read parts of that same letter, without reprimand.[15]

Hmmm, what's different about Senator Warren, compared to Senators Udall, Brown, Sanders, and Merkley? Like Udall and Brown, she's the senior senator from her state; like Sanders, she's a New Englander. Is she the only one with a law degree? No, Udall is a lawyer, too; that can't be it.

It's a head scratcher.

Whatever McConnell's motivation, women heard his words and recognized the ways they, too, had been silenced. "Nevertheless, she persisted" instantly became a rallying cry for women everywhere who had been told to sit down and shut up. The quote began a storm of social media and blog posts associating #shepersisted with Malala Yousafzai, Rosa Parks, Sonia Soto-mayor, Tammy Duckworth, Laverne Cox, and many other women who had faced adversity of all kinds and ultimately thrived.[16]

It resonated so powerfully because persisting is what women do, each and every day. Often we persist because we literally have no choice. We have children to feed and a world to change, and we can't stop just because it's hard. Overcoming obstacles like the Mitch McConnells of the world isn't just a necessary step on the way to our goals; overcoming those obstacles is part of our success! Yay!

But raise your hand if it gets exhausting. Raise your hand if you've wanted to quit. Raise your hand if you've asked yourself, *How much more do I have to do before I've done enough? How much of myself do I have to give? How smoothly do I have to polish myself before I can move through the world without friction?*

Us too.

Women's difficulty is rarely lack of persistence—on the con-trary. We stand gazing at the possibilities of what the world can be—what *we* can be. Our world can be fair; our communities can be safe; our homes can be tidy; our children can put their shoes on when it's time for school! But there is a deep, wide chasm between us and the realization of those possibilities. Our default action in the face of that chasm is to do whatever it takes to get to the other side, and keep on doing it, no matter what, until we get there.

But then we get exhausted and we wonder if we can accom-plish any of the things we hope for, without destroying ourselves in the process. We ask ourselves if it's time to quit.

Life is rarely perfect. Nearly always, there is a gap between how things are and how we wish, hope, expect, or plan for them to be. The quality of our lives is not measured by the amount of time we spend in a state of perfection. On the contrary, people of vision—think of the principal social justice leaders of the twentieth and twenty-first centuries—see the *largest* gap between what is and what ought to be, and they know they will not live to see a world that fully achieves their vision of what's possible. A gap between reality and perfection is not abnormal or a sign of dysfunction; it's a normal part of life. In fact, as we've seen, the Monitor *thrives* when things are a little frustrating, when there's always some fresh challenge, some new skill to develop, some unknown territory to chart. The quality of our lives, day to day, is measured by our freedom to choose to stay or leave. That freedom comes when we have abundance enough and safety enough to let go of what is broken and reach for something new.[17]

> *Sophie's strategy of monetizing her expertise is planful problem-solving and positive reappraisal at its most pragmatic. Is the world insisting you be good at something you never chose to be good at? Turn it into a business opportunity that solves the problem!*
>
> *People of color, women, people with disabilities, and members of other disenfranchised groups have persisted in the face of impossible frustrations, often crediting their most difficult trials with their most empowering personal growth.*
>
> *What keeps us striving when we know that we, ourselves, won't see the changes we're fighting for? Why do we persist when we hope only to make life better for the next generation?*
>
> *The answer to those questions is "meaning beyond ourselves." That science is the subject of the next chapter.*

A goal is not a life—but it may be what gives shape and direction to the way we live each day. If our goals are *what* we want to accomplish, "meaning" is *why* we want to accomplish them. We continue to do our best raising a child, even when that child makes us consider running away to join the circus. We persist at a frustrating job because we know we're making a difference in people's lives. We pursue our art, even when we know we may never make a living at it, because we simply would not be fully ourselves if we stopped. Though your goals may differ from ours, they share a common, overarching theme: they give us a sense of engagement with something larger than ourselves.

## tl;dr:

- Frustration happens when our progress toward a goal feels more effortful than we expect it to be.

- You can manage frustration by using planful problem-solving for stressors you can control, and positive reappraisal for stressors you can't control.

- When we're struggling, we may reach a point of oscillating between frustrated rage and helpless despair. Solution: Choose the right time to give up, which might be now or might be never; either way, the choice puts you back in the driver's seat.

- Your brain has a built-in mechanism to assess when it's time to quit. Listen to its quiet voice. Or do a worksheet; sometimes that's easier.

**REDEFINE WINNING**

To cope with the frustration of trying to achieve a goal that's all but impossible—e.g., "perfection"—or else eternally in-progress—e.g., "successfully" parenting a child—start by redefining what it means to "win" at this goal.

Frustrating Goal

_____

_____

What is it about this goal that frustrates your Monitor? Is it unattainable? Do you feel ambivalent about it? Was it someone else's dumb idea? Is there part of it that makes you feel helpless? Are there too many frustrating yet unavoidable obstacles between you and "winning"?

Brainstorm at least twenty options for definitions of "winning" that will satisfy your Monitor. Make sure you have plenty of silly, impractical ideas, as well as a few that could actually work. Brainstorming works best when you don't filter! For some people, it also works better when you collaborate; if that's you, ask a friend to help.

Now choose your three favorites and score them based on the criteria for Monitor-pleasing goals:

**Soon:** When will you know you've succeeded? Your goal should be achievable without requiring patience.

**Certain:** How confident are you that you can succeed? Your goal should be within your control.

**Positive:** What improvement will you experience when you win? It should be something that feels good, not just something that avoids suffering.

**Concrete:** Measurable. How will you know you've succeeded? There is an external indication that you have succeeded.

**Specific:** As opposed to general. You should be able to visualize precisely what success will look like.

**Personal:** Why does this goal matter to you? How much does it matter? Tailor your goal so that it matters to you.

|   | SOON | CERTAIN | POSITIVE | CONCRETE | SPECIFIC | PERSONAL |
|---|------|---------|----------|----------|----------|----------|
| 1. |      |         |          |          |          |          |
| 2. |      |         |          |          |          |          |
| 3. |      |         |          |          |          |          |

Reread your description of what made this goal frustrating. Now you can select whichever new definition of "winning" best addresses those problems!

# 3

# MEANING

*Some time after Julie's chocolate cake meltdown, she invited Amelia over, because, she said, she had some venting to do.*

*But instead of talking, Julie was binge-watching British children's television. It was hypnotically soothing. She stared numbly at the screen, then as the credits rolled and the music played, she said, "Jeremy's been sleeping on the couch for a week. I have no idea what might happen next." Amelia's jaw dropped, but Julie quickly added, "I don't want to talk about it."*

*They watched another fourteen-minute episode in silence. The credits ran. The TV went dark and silent and a message appeared on the screen, asking Julie if she was still watching.*

*"Don't judge me!" she yelled at the TV, and she clicked yes.*

*A third hypnotically soothing episode, and then Julie said, "I had food poisoning once. Bad. Like, sitting on the toilet with a trash can on my lap bad, you know?"*

*Wincing a little, Amelia said, "And this feels like that?"*

*Julie shook her head. "It's so much worse. Because with food poisoning you know why it's happening. You can accept it, because you know why."*

*That's the power of meaning. We can tolerate any suffering, if we know why.*

*And not knowing why is, itself, a profound type of suffering.*

*"I wrote a list," Julie said, handing Amelia a piece of paper covered in writing.*

*It was a list of questions, including,* Is this worth it? Do I want it to be worth it? *Should* it be worth it? How can I respect myself, if I give up? How can I respect myself, if I can't let go? What kind of person am I? What is love? What matters?

*"Let's watch another episode." She clicked the remote control at the TV and the colorful, singsong critters moved around the screen.*

*"I'd like to know the answer to some of these questions," Amelia interrupted. She looked at the paper and read, "What matters?"*

*How to answer that question is the subject of this chapter.*

Every Disney heroine has an "I Want" song, in which they explain what's missing in their lives. Moana feels called by the ocean. Tiana is "Almost There," saving money to start her own restaurant. Belle wants "adventure in the great wide somewhere."

The tradition goes all the way back to Snow White, singing "Someday My Prince Will Come." You can chart the progress of women in America by the things Disney heroines sing about in their "I Want" songs.

Though what they sing about changes, there is one constant: a heroine feels called by something.

Now, just as most of us do not spontaneously burst into song (though some of us do—Amelia), most of us don't lead lives of epic heroism and high-stakes adventure. We aren't chosen by the ocean to find the demigod Maui, restore the heart of Te Fiti, and save the world—nor, frankly, would most of us want to, given the choice. We've got other things on our plates. We have jobs and school. We have kids to feed, a bathtub to scrub, and an inbox to clear, not to mention novels to read and movies to watch.

But like all heroines, we thrive when we are answering the call of something larger than ourselves, when all the commuting and laundry and picking up dog poop and repeating "No television until you finish your homework!" has a *meaning* larger than the grind of daily routine.

Over the last thirty years, science has established that "meaning in life" is good for us, the way leafy green vegetables and exercise and sleep are good for us.

This chapter is about "meaning" as a power you carry inside you that helps you resist and recover from burnout. A woman's need for "meaning in life" is not fundamentally different from a man's, but the obstacles that stand between women and their sense of meaning *are* different.

## What Is It, Exactly?

Art, orgasms, and meaning in life: you probably recognize them when you encounter them, they're different from everything else, and no two people's experiences of them are exactly the same.[1]

Researchers approach "meaning" in two different ways. Positive psychology, as spearheaded by Martin Seligman, includes "Meaning" as one of the main elements that promote happiness in people who are otherwise healthy.[2] Other research approaches meaning as a coping strategy for people who are recovering from illness or trauma.[3] These different views of "meaning" have four things in common:

First, both approaches agree that meaning isn't always "fun."[4] In the happiness-enhancing approach, "meaningful" activities are described as ones "seeking to use and develop the best in oneself," in contrast to those devoted solely to "seeking pleasure."[5] In the trauma-healing model, "meaning" includes learning to "live with" chronic illness. In the first case, it's like getting your nutrients from vegetables; in the second, it's like getting nutritents through a painful but effective injection. Most of us would prefer the veggies, but sometimes the injection is our only choice.

Second, both approaches agree that meaning offers a "positive final value that an individual's life can exhibit."[6] That is, a life has meaning when a person contributes something positive to the world by the time they die—whether they enjoyed it or not. Meaning is the feeling that you "matter in some larger sense. Lives may be experienced as meaningful when they are felt to have significance beyond the trivial or momentary, to have purpose, or to have a coherence that transcends chaos."[7]

Third, meaning is not constant. Some moments in our lives feel intensely meaningful. Others feel "meaning-neutral"—you're just running errands or doing chores and it doesn't matter whether you feel a connection with something larger than yourself. Still others include a strong sense of its absence, moments when we are *seeking* meaning. We might go too long without experiencing a sense of meaning and we begin to wonder what life even *means,* or maybe terrible things happen that seem to strip life of all meaning and we ask *why.* Meaning comes and goes.

And finally, whether it supports thriving or sustains coping, meaning is good for you.[8] People with greater senses of meaning and purpose in life experience better health and are more likely to access preventative healthcare services, to protect that health.[9] A meta-analysis of the relationship between "purpose in life" and health found that greater sense of purpose was associated with a 17 percent lower risk of all-cause mortality.[10] And these benefits can be gained through active intervention. People who participate in meaning-centered psychotherapy develop greater overall well-being, relationships, and hope, as well as reduced psychological stress and improved physical health.[11] Even among people living with advanced or end-of-life disease, interventions that enhanced meaning in life had benefits for participants' depression, anxiety, distress, and overall quality of life.[12]

"Meaning," in short, is the nourishing experience of feeling like we're connected to something larger than ourselves. It helps us thrive when things are going well, and it helps us cope when things go wrong in our lives.

So, where does it come from?

## You Make It

You may be used to hearing about meaning as something we "search for" or "discover," and sometimes people experience it that way—as a sudden revelation that descends on them from on high, or a treasure that they find after years of following the map. But rarely is meaning something that we find at the end of a long, hard journey. For most of us, meaning is what sustains us on the long, hard journey, no matter what we find at the end. Meaning is not found; it is *made*.[13]

To make meaning, the research tells us, engage with something larger than yourself.[14]

This "Something Larger"—like a God you believe in or a dream you have for the future—is your source of meaning. Its mere existence is not enough, any more than the mere existence of green vegetables is enough for you to be nourished by them. You have to engage with it actively. Eat your greens. Engage with your Something Larger. Like vegetables, your Something Larger may not be the most fun thing on your plate, but it's probably the most nourishing. Unlike vegetables, you may have a sense of *calling* to engage with this Something Larger, the way heroines are called by adventure, by starting their own restaurants, or by the ocean.

Research has found that meaning is most likely to come from three kinds of sources:[15]

> 1. pursuit and achievement of ambitious goals that leave a legacy—as in "finding a cure for HIV" or "making the world a better place for these kids";
>
> 2. service to the divine or other spiritual calling—as in "attaining spiritual liberation and union with Akal" or "glorifying God with my words, thoughts, and deeds"; and
>
> 3. loving, emotionally intimate connection with others—as in "raising my kids so they know they're loved, no matter what" or "loving and supporting my partner with authenticity and kindness."

Many sources of meaning are a combination of all three, and if your Something Larger falls outside these three categories, that's cool, too. In terms of your personal well-being, there is no right or wrong source of meaning; there's just whatever gives you the feeling that your life has a positive impact.[16]

## What's Your Something Larger?

Some people know exactly what their Something Larger is, and others take years to figure it out. Amelia has always known, even when she didn't know she knew. She has wanted to be a choral conductor since she was twelve, and here she is, with three degrees in leading choral ensembles and an impressive résumé of conducting gigs. Emily stumbled from school to work to school again until, looking back to trace the pattern of the doors she had walked through, she finally figured it out, about twenty years after Amelia. Emily's Something Larger: teaching women to live with confidence and joy inside their bodies. Amelia's: art. There are plenty of other ways we could contribute—there is no end of need in the world—but these make us feel that we are contributing something positive to the world. Which is how we make meaning.

Our experiences discovering the sources of meaning in our lives might suggest there is no predictable way for each individual to find it for themselves. But the common thread is an inner voice that you can hear if you stop and listen. Everyone has it.

Hear that? The steady rhythm in the center of your chest?

Or maybe it's a slower pulse lower down, somewhere in the swell of your belly. Or a halo of wisdom crowning your skull. Stop for a minute—literally stop reading, maybe even set a timer—and listen. Ask yourself, *What am I doing when I feel most powerfully that I'm doing what I'm meant to be doing?*

Dolores Hart was a movie star with a gift for listening to that voice with what she calls "the ear of the heart." In 1964, she had starred in several major motion pictures, played a leading lady to Elvis Presley, and was starring in a Broadway play when she visited the Abbey of Regina Laudis in Bethlehem, Connecticut, for a rest. At the age of twenty-four, she was a rising star with everything the world valued most: beauty, professional success and prestige, money, and a handsome fiancé. But she had been feeling like something was wrong, something was missing.

As soon as she set foot on the abbey grounds, she felt like she had come home. Not long after, she took her vows and committed her life to God's service. She describes it:

> *In a sense, I never really felt like a person until I came to Regina Laudis. Staying was not a compromise, but, in fact, the real challenge of my life. . . . I had not chosen to escape my responsibilities by secluding myself from reality. I believed that if there is to be an ultimate and real salvation for the whole of mankind, it must begin by a very personal involvement.*[17]

She didn't enter the abbey because Catholicism offered a set of answers she preferred. Even as an inmate of a Roman Catholic monastic community, she says, "I am not easily persuaded by religious answers. . . . I have found my answers step by step."

If you're still struggling to recognize your Something Larger, research has found a few strategies that can help:

Try writing your own obituary or a "life summary" through the eyes of a grandchild or a student.

Ask your closest friends to describe the "real you," the characteristics of your personality and your life that are at the core of your best self.

Imagine that someone you care about is going through a dark moment in their life—they've experienced significant loss and feel helpless and isolated (the two things that drain us of meaning fastest). As your best self, write that person a letter to support them through this difficult time. Then reread it. It's for you.[18]

Finally, think of a time when you experienced an intense sense of meaning or purpose or "alignment" or whatever it feels like for you. What were you doing? What was it that created that sense of meaning?

All these approaches can help you distinguish your inner voice's genuine sense of Something Larger from the thing that gets in the way—namely, Human Giver Syndrome.

## Human Giver Syndrome

In the introduction, we described philosopher Kate Manne's language of "human givers" versus "human beings," a cultural code in which human beings have a moral obligation to *be* their whole humanity, while human givers have a moral obligation to *give* their whole humanity, and give it cheerfully. We call the behavior patterns associated with these moral convictions "Human Giver Syndrome."

Think of Human Giver Syndrome as a virus whose only goal is to perpetuate its own existence. You were infected with it as soon as you were born, inhaling it with your very first breath. And, just as the rabies virus makes dogs aggressive and bovine spongiform encephalopathy makes cows "mad," Human Giver Syndrome changes human behavior in order to perpetuate itself—even if it kills the host (that's us) in the process.

Do you suffer from Human Giver Syndrome? Symptoms include

- believing you have a moral obligation—that is, you *owe it* to your partner, your family, the world, or even to yourself—to be pretty, happy, calm, generous, and attentive to the needs of others;

- believing that any failure to be pretty, happy, calm, generous, and attentive makes you a failure as a person;

- believing that your "failure" means you deserve punishment—even going so far as to beat yourself up; and

- believing these are not symptoms, but normal and true ideas.

That last one is the crux, of course. What makes this metaphorical "virus" so successful as an infectious agent is that its symptoms are self-masking. It blinds you to its presence and is self-perpetuating—that is, we are surrounded by people who are also "infected," and they, too, treat themselves and us and everyone as if Human Giver Syndrome were just normal human behavior, which reinforces our own sense that it is not a disease at all, but a healthy, normal way to live.

If you were raised in a culture shaped by Human Giver Syndrome, you were taught to prioritize being pretty, happy, calm, generous, and attentive to the needs of others, above anything else. Maybe—*maybe*—you can pursue your own personal (read: selfish) Something Larger, if you've thoroughly met the needs of everyone else and don't stop being pretty and calm while you do it.

On the surface, Human Giver Syndrome seems to support some Something Largers, like *being of service*. Service is what givers are supposed to do anyway, and it is a defining characteristic of the great figures of history.

Audre Lorde: "When I dare to be powerful, to use my strength in the service of my vision, then it becomes less and less important whether I am afraid."[19]

Malala Yousafzai: "I raise up my voice—not so I can shout, but so that those without a voice can be heard."

Shirley Chisholm: "Service to others is the rent you pay for your room here on earth."

Hillary Clinton: "Do all the good you can, for all the people you can, in all the ways you can, for as long as you can."[20]

But each one of these women worked to be "of service" in ways that violated their roles as human givers. And if you do that—say, by leaving someone else's needs unmet, or not being pretty and calm while you do it, or claiming power that "rightfully" belongs not to a human giver but to a human being—the world smacks you down.

They say, "What's the matter with you?"

They say, "Get back in line."

This is a theme we'll encounter over and over through the rest of this book: Behave yourself. Follow the rules. Or else.

Human Giver Syndrome goes so far as to insist we're wrong to see ourselves as heroines battling an enemy. A giver has no needs and thus has nothing to fight for. Joseph Campbell himself, father of the "Hero's Journey" framework, summarized it succinctly when presented with a "Heroine's Journey" to consider. He said, "Women don't need to make the journey. In the whole mythological journey, the woman is there. All she has to do is realize she's the place people are trying to get to."[21]

Women are a "place"; only men are "people" on a journey, with a villain to defeat. Women's Something Larger is men.

Tell that to Malala; lots of people did. Tell it to U.S. Representative Tammy Duckworth, who lost her legs in combat during the Iraq War and then became the first disabled woman and among the first Asian American women elected to the U.S. Congress. Tell it to Tona Brown, the first out transwoman of color to play Carnegie Hall. Tell it to Ellen Ochoa, the first Latina to go to space and now the director of the Johnson Space Center. Tell it to every woman who ever worked a soul-eroding factory job or cleaned other people's houses eighty hours a week or danced at a strip club, all to pay the bills, to keep the heat on, so her kids wouldn't be cold at night—or to get an education, to become a leader in her discipline.

Tell her, "What's wrong with you? Get back in line. You don't need to go anywhere; you just need to be the place a man is trying to get to."

We say it all the time, to other women and to ourselves. To suffer from Human Giver Syndrome is to be convinced, on some level, that everyone should suffer along with us. And so if we see someone who looks like they're not even trying, we feel outraged. When we see women who aren't trying to control their appearance or their emotions so that they aren't making anyone uncomfortable, or who use their time, money, and labor to improve their own well-being rather than someone else's, "What's the matter with her?" we say to ourselves. "If I have to follow the rules, so does she! She needs to *get back in line*." And we call that unruly woman fat or bossy or full of herself. As if those are bad things.

In a sense, Human Giver Syndrome is the first villain in our story. It tries to make you ignore your Something Larger, because you're supposed to dedicate all your resources to Human Beings. But how can we escape or defeat the villain in our own story when we're busy policing others to keep them from defeating it?

The good news is, when you engage with your Something Larger and thus make meaning in your life, you're actually healing Human Giver Syndrome, both in yourself and in the people around you.

## Make Meaning, Heal Human Giver Syndrome

Human Giver Syndrome used to tell women that their place— their *only* place—was in the home (and in some places, it still does). Betty Friedan documented how *giving* was weaponized to manipulate housewives of the 1950s and '60s, forcing them away from the workplace they had inhabited during the Second World War by insisting that homemaking was the (only) Something Larger that would fulfill them as women. And if, as Betty Freidan so memorably put it, they didn't "have an orgasm waxing the kitchen floor,"[22] it wasn't anyone's fault but their own. If homemaking left them unfulfilled or dissatisfied, then they were broken as women. Until Freidan named this "problem that has no name," millions of women had been suffering in silence.

The second-wave feminist movement created a new force that allowed women to push for something different or just more and not be asked, "What's the matter with you?" It opened up new possibilities for women. It motivated personal life changes and political action and a cultural shift that, in turn, changed the culture itself.

There was backlash—there always is. Human Giver Syndome

punishes those who try to treat it, and many paid a price for their resistance or rebellion. But the long-term result was an incrementally fairer world.

Human Giver Syndrome will try to stop you from pursuing meaning. Your job is to not stop. Keep engaging with your Something Larger. Use planful problem-solving. Keep completing the cycle. #Persist.

But of course, sometimes it's not that easy.

*Sophie engages with her Something Larger—SCIENCE FOR ALL!—in many different ways. Her work, of course, is one way. Her mentoring of young women in STEM is another. Her consulting and speaking about making STEM more welcoming for women of color is still another. She works extremely hard, many hours a day, in environments that are often pretty toxic, and she makes a real difference in the world. Hundreds of people could tell you how she has changed their lives for the better.*

*Sophie's Star Trek fandom is her most playful source of meaning. When she was a little girl, Sophie saw Lieutenant Uhura on TV and knew that she could be a black girl and a scientist and an explorer and be taken seriously. And because she saw that it was possible, she believed nothing could stand between her and that goal.*

*And what is she now? An engineer.*

*Sophie's a hardcore fan. She even has an Uhura costume—not a Zoe Saldana Uhura costume, or even a 1979 Star Trek: The Motion Picture beige jumpsuit, but a season three minidress, as worn by Nichelle Nichols, scoop collar, bracelet sleeves, and all, in engineering red. She wears it to Star Trek conventions, where she connects with fellow fans who dwell with her in an optimistic future where anyone can be an engineer, an explorer. For her, cosplay is practice living inside a world where that future already exists.*

*And in a way, it does already exist—in her. From the pointed toes of her mid-calf boots to the top of her bouffant wig, Sophie is six feet five inches of everything* Star Trek *aspired to—and of the vision Dr. Martin Luther King, Jr., shared when he convinced Nichelle Nichols to stay in the role of Lieutenant Uhura.[23] As Nichols tells the story, "For the first time, we are being seen by the world over as we should be seen. [King] says, 'Do you understand that this is the only show that my wife Coretta and I will allow our little children to stay up and watch?'"*

*Making the world a better place for all scientists is not just patient explanations of what privilege is and stories of "accidental" exclusion of women and people of color. It can also be a bright red minidress and winged eyeliner. When Sophie climbs out of her car at a Trekker convention and hands her keys to the valet, every human turns to look and admire. Everyone wants to take pictures with her.*

*And when they find out she is an actual, real-life engineer, many times their brains turn inside out.*

*Uhura's first name is Nyota, the Swahili word for "star."*

*As in, what we reach for.*

## Making Meaning When Terrible Things Happen

When life is stable, we don't need much sense of meaning to stay well. We engage regularly with our Something Larger, and our brains metabolize those experiences to keep us feeling like the world makes sense and our existence has purpose. Hooray!

But.

Sometimes life gets rocky.

When an airplane bounces into a sudden pocket of turbulence, you grab the arms of your seat, as if by holding your seat, you can hold the plane steady. You, of course, know it doesn't work that way, but your hands don't. They will hold on to anything they can reach, and the very fact of holding on makes the turbulence more tolerable.

When our lives bounce through pockets of turbulence—such as the uncertainty of joblessness or a confrontation with death or a sense that our work is not making a difference or that we don't belong—our brains grab hold of our Something Larger, as if it can stop our lives or the world from tumbling out of the sky. And it works.[24] It helps us tolerate the uncertainty, the mortality, the helplessness or loneliness, until we find ourselves on the other side of the turbulence and back in smooth airspace.

But sometimes the turbulence lasts too long, or the plane actually crashes. You survive, but you're left in an "existential vacuum," devoid of meaning.[25] Terrible things happen, leaving us feeling trapped and convinced that nothing we do can make a difference. In such times of crisis, we have to repair the plane before we can return to our journey. That requires us to turn inward toward difficult feelings with kindness and compassion.

Those Disney princess "I Want" stories each have a point where our heroine is in crisis and has to stop and take time to turn inward. Moana has to repair her boat. Snow White needs a long nap and a kiss from her true love. Tiana is forced to stop pursuing her dream when she is turned into a frog; solving the frog problem by "digging a little deeper" not only allows her to get closer to her dream, but also makes her a princess. With compassion for the wounded parts of our hearts, minds, bodies, and communities, our recovery from adversity can include an *increased* sense of meaning in life, moving us from coping to thriving.

Example: A study of more than three thousand U.S. veterans who had all experienced trauma found that those experiencing post-traumatic stress disorder (PTSD) symptoms were more likely than those without PTSD to experience post-traumatic *growth*. This included both a better sense of personal strength

("I discovered that I'm stronger than I thought I was" and "I know better that I can handle difficulties") and appreciation of life ("I have a greater appreciation for the value of my own life").[26]

How do they do it? How can people continue to engage with their Something Larger even in the face of terrible things? Even in the face of terrible things that separate them from their Something Larger?

The key is: You can never be separated from your Something Larger, because it is inside you.

---

### ORIGIN STORY

Want to turn something terrible into an unlooked-for opportunity to engage with your Something Larger and make meaning? Rewrite the narrative of your experience, focusing on the lessons and strengths you gained through adversity.[27] We call this your "origin story," like the origin of Batman's life as a superhero in the tragic death of his parents or the origin of Wonder Woman on the sheltered shores of Themyscira.

Take half an hour or so to write your story, answering these questions:

1. **What parts of the adversity were uncontrollable by you? (e.g., other people and their choices, cultural norms, your life circumstances at the time, your age and prior experience, the weather...)**

2. **What did you do to survive the adversity, in the moment? (Hint: We know for sure that you did successfully survive the adversity, because here you are.)**

**3. What resources did you leverage, to continue surviving after the adversity had passed?** Be specific. (May include practical resources, like money or information; social resources like friends, your ability to seek, find, and accept help, or your social influence; or emotional resources like persistence, self-soothing, and optimism.)

Once you have your story, take a moment to write about a time when those resources empowered you to overcome a subsequent difficulty.

Then write a summary:

Even though I couldn't control _____ (adversity), I managed to _____ (survival tactic), and then I used _____ (resource) to grow stronger. After that, I could _____ (skill/win/insight).

Writing an origin story can even help you identify your Something Larger, because it helps you notice the parts of your past experience that you leveraged to survive.[28] Meaning is not made by the terrible thing you experienced; it is made by the ways you survive.

This process might hurt. That's actually another part of what makes this practice effective: It allows your body to practice feeling the feelings of past wounds, to learn that those feelings are not dangerous, and to complete the incomplete stress response cycles activated all those years ago.[29] It starts with your willingness to look, to risk the discomfort of paying attention to what you thought was only negative, and to learn to see it with nonjudgment, curiosity, and even compassion.

## Your Something Larger Is Within You

Moana's Something Larger is the ocean; she feels it calling her. As she tells Maui, the ocean *chose* her for her mission. Almost no one agrees with her. Her family wants her to stay home and be chief of her island. Maui is skeptical that the ocean would choose "a curly-haired non-princess" who can't sail. Then some terrible things happen and Moana drops into the pit of despair. She even tells the ocean to "choose someone else."

But the ghost of her grandmother, the "village crazy lady" who always believed in her, appears and nudges Moana to remember who she is. As Moana considers what has brought her to this pivotal moment, she realizes (in song form): "The call isn't out there at all / It's inside me!"

The call was never coming from "out there"; it was coming from inside her own heart. She was the "chosen one" not because something outside her chose her and called across a distance, but because something in her own heart was calling, and so, without even knowing it, she chose herself.

"Moana" is the Maori word for "ocean"; Disney made the lesson nice and literal.

Whatever calls you, whether it's the ocean or art or family or democracy, isn't out there. It's inside you. Like all the cycles and rhythms we describe in this book, it comes and goes, accelerates and decelerates, falls away and rises again. Like a tide, inside you. But no matter what forces oppose you, whether it's Human Giver Syndrome or natural disasters or personal loss, nothing can stand between you and your Something Larger.

Your Something Larger lives inside you. Maybe everyone around you disagrees. Maybe your family wants you to stay home—or leave home. Maybe even your mentors are skeptical, and only the village crazy lady agrees with you. Still, you hear it over the noise of Human Giver Syndrome and through the suffering of violence and injustice. *You* know; you hear the call in your heart.

*Julie breathed deeply and stared in the direction of the TV, pondering the question of what matters to her. "My daughter definitely matters," she said, fluids dripping from most of the orifices in her face. "Diana. Teaching is so important, you know, it really matters, but even if I lost that, if I lost everything else, it would be okay as long as I had Diana."*

*And she cried for a long time, until the truth started hurting less.*

*And that was enough—that moment, that reminder—to get her through a little more of the most challenging time of her life.*

*"I just need a little more help," she said at last. "We'd been having this same fight over and over and he wasn't hearing me and nothing had changed. I just couldn't do it anymore. I ran out of 'can.' I lost the ability to can. If I do everything, if I manage his feelings and the house and everything, then I'm exhausted. And if I don't do it, I suffer from his shitty mood and nothing gets done. I'm just tired. When I made him move downstairs, I didn't even have the energy to be mad, you know? I was too tired to yell."*

*She wasn't where she needed to be yet, to preserve her own well-being. It would take a more blatant wake-up call to force her to turn and fight for larger-scale, longer-term well-being. But sometimes it's enough just to get through the day and still feel like there's a reason to keep struggling.*

During World War II, an unknown Jew, hiding from the Nazis, scratched these words into the wall of a cellar:[30]

> *I believe in the sun, even when it is not shining.*
> *I believe in love, even when feeling it not.*
> *I believe in God, even when He is silent.*

This is not a poem that explains what the Holocaust might "mean." How can genocide ever "mean" anything to its victims and survivors? It's a poem about how a person can make it through such horrors. We can't "believe" our way out of oppression, exile, or despair. But when we make meaning, we can sustain ourselves through worse things than we can imagine.

"Meaning in life" is made when you engage with the Something Larger that's waiting for you inside your own body, linking you to the world. It doesn't take much, but it's important because our "meaning in life," established when we're doing well, will be a bedrock to support us, whatever adversity we face. We can hold on, come what may, by listening to the quietness inside ourselves, that knows the world makes sense.

There is plenty of adversity in the world, and it's the topic of the next two chapters. But we want you to confront it knowing you are well armed with these innate weapons and the skill to use them. You've got your stress response and the knowledge of how to complete the cycle. You've got your Monitor and planful problem-solving and positive reappraisal. You've got your Something Larger. They will protect you from adversity. They will heal you in the aftermath of adversity.

So this is the point in the story where we step away from the shelter of internal experience. This is the time when we stand and look into the face of the enemy.

It's about to get pretty dark. But you're ready.

## tl;dr:

- "Meaning in life" is good for you. You make meaning by engaging with something larger than yourself—whether that's ambitious goals, service to the divine, or loving relationships.

- Meaning enhances well-being when you're doing well, and it can save your life when you're struggling.

- Human Giver Syndrome is a collection of personal and cultural beliefs and behaviors that insist that some people's only "meaning in life" comes from being pretty, happy, calm, generous, and attentive to the needs of others.

- The stress response cycle, the Monitor, and meaning are all resources you carry with you into the battle against the real enemy.

# PART II

## The Real Enemy

# 4

# THE GAME IS RIGGED

*Sophie was taking her show on the road, being paid—
a lot—to speak at corporate meetings about creating
workplaces that support a diverse workforce. She was running some drafts of her talk by Emily, for her pedagogical
expertise.*

*"What's that?" Emily asked, pointing to an unfamil-
iar word on a PowerPoint slide.*

*"Kobayashi Maru," Sophie said, and when Emily
looked blank, she explained, "It's a training simulation
for Starfleet cadets, an unwinnable scenario designed to
test your character. You can't win, so the goal is to lose in
a way that's honorable."*

*"A Star Trek thing?" Emily asked.*

*"A Star Trek thing," Sophie confirmed, "that turns*

*systemic bias into a game." She clicked to the next slide. "People hire people they know, people who went to the same schools." She pointed to the statistics graphic, then clicked to the next slide, which was full of references to Implicit Associations research. "They have an unconscious bias that makes them prefer people who look like them." The next slide was covered in images from movies, TV shows, videogames, and comic books. "Every piece of media they consume affirms their biases. And"—she clicked to the next slide, which was covered in dozens of characters, all white, all men, all heroes: knights in shining armor, men in capes, mutants with telepathic abilities, wizards, detectives, wizard detectives—"they see that spaces filled with white men are not just normal, but better."*

*Her tone lightened to her more usual geeky excitement. "So here I am, trying to rescue the ship in the Neutral Zone, and the Klingons are going to attack. I. Am. Going. To. Die. The win is I prove my character every time I'm tested."*

*"You're going to tell them outright that they're creating an unwinnable scenario?"*

*Sophie nodded. "The science says it's good for us to name it."*

*That science is the subject of this chapter.*

In the wake of violence, the first priority is to stop the bleeding and save the victim's life. But at some point, we need to go back and figure out how the bleeding started so we can prevent it from happening again. We need to talk about the knife and the person who used it against us.

The tools we described in Part I stop the bleeding; they can help you right now. They can quite literally save your life. Every human can complete the stress response cycle, manage their Monitor, and engage with their Something Larger, because those resources exist inside us. You'll have access to them all your life, no matter where you go, no matter what culture you live in.

But we need to talk about where the bleeding came from—the knife, and the enemy who wielded it.

If you're a woman in the industrialized West, you'll confront a particular set of enemies that will try to cut you down to size, over and over, and they'll lie to your face while they do it, saying it's for your own good, saying you should be grateful for their "help." And because we've been confronting these enemies literally since before we were born, we often believe them.

To explain, we need to talk about some rat research. We promise it's worth it.

Okay: Imagine two rats. Rat #1—let's call him Ralph the Rat . . . only pronounced "Rafe," like Ralph Fiennes. In fact, let's say it's not a rat, it is actually Ralph Fiennes. He's in a box—it's called a "shuttle box"—with a floor that periodically electrocutes his feet. It's not painful, but it is uncomfortable. Ralph hates being electrocuted and he wants to get out of there every time it happens. Fortunately for him, after the zapping begins, a little door opens briefly, and he can make a run for it! He escapes! His dopamine levels double, as his Monitor quickly learns that escaping the shock is an attainable goal! He has overcome adversity and learned that he can make a difference in his situation.

Rat #2—we'll call him Colin—and let's make it Colin Firth, because why not?—is not in a box; he's in a tank of water, for the "forced-swim test." (You can tell it's bad just by the name, right?) Colin, like most rats, can swim—he did it in *Pride and Prejudice* and *A Single Man*—but he doesn't love it; he'd like to get out of the water as soon as possible. So he swims and swims and swims and swims . . . and never reaches dry land. As he keeps failing, he get frustrated . . . and then desperate! Foopy! And ultimately Colin's Monitor switches its assessment of his goal from "potentially attainable" to "unattainable." His dopamine levels drop by half; he feels helpless, and he just floats, in a last-ditch effort to reserve energy until there's any sign of land.

Here's maybe the saddest part about this: If we take Colin out of the water, dry him off, and put him into the shuttle box, he will not even try to escape the shock, though the door is right there.[1] In the shuttle box, Colin could escape if he tried, but he *can't* try. His brain has learned that trying doesn't work, that nothing he does makes a difference . . . and so he has lost the ability to try.

This inability to try is called "learned helplessness." Animals, including humans, who repeatedly find themselves in bad situations from which they can't escape may not even *try* to escape, even when given the opportunity. When an animal has learned helplessness, it goes straight past frustration right to the pit of despair. It's not a rational choice; their central nervous system has learned that when they are suffering, nothing they can do will make a difference. They have learned they are helpless. Their only available route for self-preservation is not to try.

When you read studies like these—and there are hundreds of them—part of you can't help wanting to go to the rat and let him in on the secret: "Colin, this thing is rigged! The experimenters are messing with you on purpose, just to see how you'll react."

That's what researchers do when they study learned helplessness in humans. In one example, researchers subjected study participants to an annoying noise that participants either could or could not turn off. Many participants in the "helpless" group shut down as the rats did, and simply stopped trying to solve the problem. But researchers made sure participants didn't walk out of the experiment trapped in the pit of despair. As soon as a participant in the "helpless" group was "shown that the noise was rigged or the problem was unsolvable, his symptoms would disappear."[2]

Just knowing that the game is rigged can help you feel better right away.

And that's what this chapter is for.

In the young adult dystopian series *The Hunger Games,* Katniss Everdeen is forced into a "game" in which she has to kill other children. It's a ritual developed by the totalitarian government to control the provinces.

Before she goes into the game, her mentor says, "Remember who the real enemy is."

We are not our own worst enemy. Nor is the enemy the other people in the game.

The enemy is *the game itself,* which tries to convince us that it's not the enemy.

Let's get started.

## The Patriarchy. (Ugh.)

We know. The word "patriarchy" makes many people uncomfortable. If you're one of those people, that's completely fine. You don't need to accept the word, or use it, to recognize the symptoms of living in it. Its messages ring inside us like a song that's been stuck in our heads so long that we don't even notice it anymore, not recognizing that it was taught to us in our infancy.

On the day a baby is born (if not sooner), the adults declare either "It's a boy!" or "It's a girl!" If no difference existed in the way boys and girls were treated, a baby's genitals would be no more important in deciding how the child was raised than any other part of their body. But instead, the baby is treated as if all sorts of other things about them are true—what kind of toys they'll enjoy, what skills they'll develop, whom they'll grow up to fall in love with, what they'll want to be when they grow up.

The difference between how boys and girls are raised is gradually shrinking; more and more, fathers are in favor of their daughters possessing "traditionally masculine" traits like "independence" and "strength" . . . even if they're not so enthusiastic about their own wives or girlfriends possessing those same characteristics. But our expectations are still widely different for girls and boys; you can see how wide the difference is simply by looking at the toy aisle for girls and the toy aisle for boys. The difference isn't neutral. Being raised as a boy makes it easier for boys to grow up and take on positions of power and authority, which is all "patriarchy" means.

This takes a lot of forms:

*Explicit misogyny.* One example of this is a reality TV star declaring he can grab women "by the pussy" whenever he wants because he's famous, and a flood of media coverage suggesting that this sort of thing is perfectly okay—"just locker-room talk." Imagine if he (or a woman) had said he can "grab men by the dick" whenever he wanted.

Or a young man goes on a murderous rampage, killing several people and injuring many more, and justifies it by saying women refuse to have sex with him. In response to one such mass murderer who identified as an "incel" ("involuntarily celibate"), *The New York Times* ran an op-ed that unjokingly argued that "redistribution of sex"—that is, sex for men, with women—was a reasonable idea.[3] You see, women could be preventing these deaths, if only they did their job of meeting the sexual needs of dangerous men.

In the time that we were writing this book, there were fifteen public mass shootings in the United States perpetrated by men or boys, several of whom were motivated, at least in part, by some form of jealousy, sexual frustration, or emotional rejection by a woman or girl.[4] In more than half of all mass shootings, the perpetrator kills his intimate partner or family members, including his mother, his wife or girlfriend, or his children.[5]

*Sex and relationship violence.* Sexual assault disproportionately and systematically targets women: women are three times more likely than men to be assaulted, while 95 percent of sex offenders are men; one in five American women college students experiences sexual assault or attempted sexual assault during college.[6] Globally, men who rape women report that their primary motivation is the basic belief that they have a right to a woman's body, regardless of how she feels about it, a belief termed "sexual entitlement" in the research.[7] Women are held responsible for being assaulted based on how they "lead men on" with behavior or attire, but perpetrators are disproportionately underprosecuted. At the same time, public officials accused of sexual assault are allowed to defend themselves by implying that the woman making the accusation is too ugly to rape.

In addition to the threat of acute physical and sexual violence, women face chronic gendered stressors every day. These experiences of patriarchy are like traffic noise in a big city. If you live there, you get so used to it you hardly notice it anymore, but that doesn't make it less noisy. The noise includes:

*Body image.* We talk about this extensively in chapter 5, so we'll save a complete discussion for then, but we want to mention now that body dysmorphia and disordered eating disproportionately and systematically impact women more than men, and the dynamic is already in place by elementary school, with half of six-year-old girls worrying they're "too fat." And let's remember that eating disorders have the highest mortality of any mental health issue. Body image isn't about vanity; women's lives are on the line.

*Getting a word in edgewise.* Again, the dynamic is already in place by elementary school: boys speak up and call out answers eight times more than girls.[8] Among grown-ups, in meetings where men are the majority, women speak a third less than men; only when there are more women than men do women speak as much as men.[9] During President Barack Obama's first term in office, his women staffers struggled so much to get their voices heard that they coordinated an "amplification" tactic, where when one of them made a key point, the others would repeat it, crediting the original speaker. Even President Obama, a self-declared feminist, needed active intervention to create gender balance.

In rat research, these kinds of pervasive problems are called "chronic, mild stress." Rats may be deprived of food and water for unpredictable—but not dangerous—periods of time; their cages tilted at a 45-degree angle for a few hours; water poured on their bedding; strobe lights flashed for hours at a time. Everything is just a little bit too hard, so that every day, bit by bit, the survivable helplessness eats away at them.[10] In human terms, researchers are creating for these rats a context of "one damn thing after another."

In the twenty-first-century West, "one damn thing after another" is what being a woman often feels like. It's a constant, low-level stream of stressors that are out of your control. Most individual examples are little more than an annoyance . . . but they accumulate.

We're not saying life isn't difficult for everyone, or that men and boys don't struggle with these issues, too. They do. The pressure to conform to an ever-shrinking mold is increasing as companies discover how much profit there is to be made from telling men they aren't valuable unless they have six-pack abs or instantaneous erections. People of every gender die in mass murders, often including the killer, and men are more likely to die by violence, including at their own hand. Misogyny doesn't just kill women.

But that's another book. We're here to address the fact that we exist in an environment where women are more likely than men to get back to their nest to find that someone has poured water on their bedding.

Womanhood as a "chronic, low-level stress" is even messier than it sounds, for two reasons: First, it's very possible that female and male biologies respond differently to that stress. When male rats are exposed to these chronic, mild stressors, their swim time in the forced swim drops in half pretty much right away. After six weeks, it drops in half again. Female rats, by contrast, take three weeks to drop their swim time in half . . . and it doesn't change after six weeks. Female rats exposed to chronic, mild stressors persist more than males do. They work harder in the face of difficulty; it takes twice as long for their brains to shift into helplessness. Even female rats, it seems, #persist.

And second, one of the stressors we experience is being told that we're not experiencing any more or different stress than men. One aspect of the patriarchy (ugh) in the modern West is that it says it doesn't exist anymore.

## Gaslighting

Remember the movie *Gaslight*? Ingrid Bergman's husband flickers the lights (gaslights, from before electricity) but tells her she's imagining it. He puts a watch in her bag and tells her she stole it. He snoops around in the attic looking for her dead aunt's jewels, and tells Ingrid she's imagining the footsteps she hears. He denies her contact with other people, saying it's for her own good because clearly her nerves are shaky.

Isolated and trapped, what can she do but believe him?

In the movie, Ingrid Bergman is finally vindicated when a policeman, dreamboat Joseph Cotten, comes to her house and says, "Yes, the gaslights are flickering. You are not crazy."

This story resonated so strongly with generations of moviegoers that "gaslighting" has become a term to describe the larger phenomenon of women and other marginalized groups being told over and over that it's their imagination.

That thing people do, when they tell you you're imagining the discrimination? They're gaslighting you.

And that feeling you have when someone is doing it to you but you're not sure because maybe they're right and you're overreacting and being too sensitive? Like you can't trust your own senses, except what your senses are telling you is unambiguous? That's feeling *gaslit*. You're filled with simultaneous doubt, fear, rage, betrayal, isolation, and panicked confusion. You can feel that a situation is wrong, but you can't explain why or how. So you worry that you misunderstood something, or you feel inadequate for being unable to articulate your objection.

It's hard to go to a friend and explain what happened, how you reacted and why. Without recognizing gaslighting for what it is, you might even hesitate to share that story at all because gaslighting is designed to make you question your own credibility and competence. But rest assured. You're not wrong or stupid: you've been gaslit.

Pundits on TV inform us that sexism isn't a thing anymore (#notallmen, and P.S.: neither is racism #alllivesmatter), so if we're not paid as much as the men (or the white people) we work with, that's because we haven't earned it—or, worse, because men ask for what they want, and if we would just ask, we would get it. And if we ask but don't get it, it's because we didn't ask the right way. Magazines tell us that if we just drink ten green smoothies a day, we'll feel great and look great, our kids will say "please" and "thank you," and our boss will give us that promotion. And if none of those things happen, it's because we failed to drink the ten green smoothies; it's certainly not because of systemic bias.

The message is consistent and persistent—whatever is wrong, *it's your fault*. It can't be true that the whole rest of the world is broken or crazy; *you're* the one who's broken and crazy. You haven't tried hard enough. You haven't done the right things. You don't have what it takes.

Eventually, what can we do but believe them?

Gaslighting creates deeply uncomfortable feelings of being trapped, while making you believe you put yourself in that trap, which just makes you angrier and sadder and less hopeful.

Some people who gaslight you are doing it on purpose.[11] They're the bully who grabs your hand and slaps you with it, chanting, "Stop hitting yourself! Stop hitting yourself!"

But not everyone who gaslights is a jerk. Some of them suffer from what we might call "patriarchy blindness." We've found two causes of this blindness: Human Giver Syndrome and the "headwinds/tailwinds asymmetry."

## Patriarchy Blindness #1: Human Giver Syndrome

At the heart of Human Giver Syndrome lies the deeply buried, unspoken assumption that women should give everything, every moment of their lives, every drop of energy, to the care of others. "Self-care" is, indeed, selfish because it uses personal resources to promote a giver's well-being, rather than someone else's.

Human Giver Syndrome is the framework on which the "second shift" hangs—the shrinking but ongoing inequality in the time and effort spent on childcare and housekeeping between men and women—forty hours per week for women versus an hour and a half for men, globally.[12] Even in the most balanced nations—which include the United States, the United Kingdom, and Canada—women still spend 50 percent more time in this unpaid labor.[13] For example, the difference was twenty-six hours per week for women, versus sixteen hours for men in the United Kingdom, in 2016.[14]

Worse, Human Giver Syndrome is the framework on which sexual violence hangs—the basic belief that men have a right to women's bodies, and if a woman looks attractive to a man or puts herself in a position where a man can take control of her body, well, that's what happens; men have a right to take what they can get. This isn't just an emotional and cultural dynamic. It has been and still is a literal, legally sanctioned reality. For millennia in the United Kingdom, a woman and everything she possessed became the legal property of the man who married her. Only recently did a woman gain the right to keep her own property when she married (1882), to keep her name (1924), and to not be raped by her husband (1991).[15]

Human Giver Syndrome is so deeply ingrained, it takes being confronted with statistics and dates to reveal the imbalances and injustice to us. Without large-scale, objective measurement and historical perspective, it's all too easy to feel comfortable with the familiar inequalities: Human givers don't own or control anything, not even their bodies, so when we hear about a woman being sexually harassed, abused, or assaulted by a man, we lament the ways an accusation of sexual assault or harassment will hinder the man's promising career, and suggest that the woman doing the accusing brought it on herself. Accusers get death threats, and the accused is put on the Supreme Court.

In short, it's easy to be blind.

So how do we keep our eyes open, and help others to see?

When we teach college students about human beings and human givers, we ask, "What's the solution?"

What do you think?

The first answer students give is nearly always, "Raise everyone to be human beings!"

Let's think about that for a second. What would a world look like in which everyone was a human being, competitive, acquisitive, and entitled?

One philosophy major, faced with this image, blurted out, "Solitary, poor, nasty, brutish, and short," quoting Thomas Hobbes, who saw the "state of nature" as a "war of all against all," because "man, whose joy consisteth in comparing himself with other men," is "continually in competition for honour and dignity."

If we raise everyone to be "human beings," the result is eternal war and/or, if we follow Hobbes, totalitarian government. Fun! And the fact that so many students automatically assume that the category "human beings"—that is, men—is the default and "human giver"—that is, women—is the alternative, is itself a symptom of Human Giver Syndrome. It is "patriarchy blindness."

Now, what if . . . just what if . . . we raised everyone to be a version of a human giver? What if we assumed it was *every* person's moral responsibility to be generous and attentive to the needs of others? What if we assumed no one was simply entitled to have what they wanted from another person, but everyone was supposed to try to help others whenever they could?

No one would sit watching television while the other cooked dinner and did the dishes, unless both had mutually agreed that what worked best for both of them was that one should rest while the other gave. No law would allow anyone to take control of another person's body, because no one would expect that right. No one would feel the mess of doubt, betrayal, sadness, and rage that comes from being gaslit, because no one would gaslight. And when anyone dropped into the pit of despair, the givers who surround them would turn toward them with generous compassion, without judgment. The absence of the patriarchy (ugh) makes being a human giver safer.

Human Giver Syndrome is deeply entrenched and it takes time and practice to eradicate it. Even after spending decades working in sexual violence prevention and response, Emily still notices periodic twinges of Human Giver Syndrome, fleeting thoughts of "Why did she go into his room?" or "Why didn't she leave?" The goal is not to eliminate these ideas entirely; it is to spot them earlier and earlier, because they're easier to uproot when they're small. To recognize when Human Giver Syndrome may be blinding her to the patriarchy, Emily uses a simple gut check. She asks herself, "How would I feel about this, if it were a man instead of a woman [or vice versa]?"

Or, "Am I assuming this woman has a moral obligation to be pretty, happy, calm, generous, or attentive to the needs of others?" and "Am I assuming this man has a moral right and obligation to be competitive and acquisitive, to take and have anything he can, regardless of the impact on others?"

Human Giver Syndrome blinds us to the patriarchy (ugh),

because it constrains our ability to view gender-based inequalities, imbalances, and injustices as unfair.

But it's not the only reason a person might be blinded.

## Patriarchy Blindness #2:
## Headwinds/Tailwinds Asymmetry

In Emily's long-distance-cycling days, she noticed that a flat part of her ride was flatter on the way home than on the way out.

"Huh?" you ask. "How could the same road be flatter going south than it was going north?"

In fact, the "flat" road had a grade of less than 1 percent above horizontal. It looked flat, but if it were actually flat, it would have felt the same in both directions, or maybe more difficult on the way home, when her legs were fatigued from the twenty-plus miles she had just ridden. Yet it felt noticeably *easier* on the way home. The strangest part is that, because it *looked* flat, her brain and her legs interpreted the sensation of zipping over the southbound road as what flat was supposed to feel like, and the difficulty of the northbound ride as somehow more difficult than flat was supposed feel.

This sort of bias is called the "headwinds/tailwinds asymmetry," because people tend to notice their adversarial headwinds and not their helpful tailwinds. It shows up in all kinds of people, in all kinds of situations. Researchers have found that Americans generally believe that the electoral college and campaign finance systems give unfair advantage to whichever political party they disagree with most, regardless of what the evidence says. People similarly believe their preferred sports team had more disadvantages going into a game than the other team. People even report that their parents were easier on their siblings than on themselves—no matter what their siblings have to say about it.[16] In so many ways, most of us tend to ignore or forget about advantages we've received, but remember the obstacles we've overcome, because the struggle against the obstacles requires more effort and energy than the easy parts.

Falling victim to headwinds/tailwinds asymmetry isn't the same as being a jerk. Jerks complain about being treated unfairly when the reality is they're being treated fairly instead of being given preferential treatment. But most of the time, when people insist, for example, that women don't have it harder than men, they're expressing headwinds/tailwinds asymmetry. When National Public Radio (NPR) covers a new study that shows male doctors are half as likely to introduce a fellow female doctor as "Dr. So-and-so,"[17] the Facebook comments in response to the story are full of women saying, "How screwed up is it that we need a study to prove what every woman knows?" and men saying, "What about teh menz?"[18] Those men aren't necessarily jerks; they're just oblivious of their tailwinds.

White people inflict their headwinds/tailwinds asymmetry on people of color all the time; the road *looks* flat, so how could it be any less flat for people of color? It must be that the brown person just isn't as strong a cyclist or they're lazy or entitled. It can't be a problem with the road. White people are not all jerks, but we are, most of us, victims of the headwinds/tailwinds asymmetry.

People from affluent families do it to poor people; citizens do it to immigrants; nondisabled people do it to people with disabilities. People in any dominant group find it impossible to believe that the road isn't as flat for others as it is for them; they only know they're working really hard. But there is a simple reality check to help counteract this cognitive bias.

*Even as Julie was wrestling with marriage difficulties, she got a new job at a high school in the same school district. It was a big improvement—better administrators, plus more money, flexibility, and prestige. On top of that, she was in charge of the theater program, which was a dream come true.*

*When Amelia emailed to ask how the new job was*

going, Julie replied: "I love it, I'm exhausted, it's amazing, my brain is thrilled, my stomach hurts. I'm so lucky. CAN YOU BELIEVE THIS: I'm the first woman ever to run the theater program at this school! WHAT? HOW."

For the first time, Julie was directing a high school theater production. She had written plays in college and had basic theater training, but had never been in charge of the whole thing the way her new job required her to be.

So many decisions had to be made, so much work had to be done. She found herself drowning in work, unable to find time to do enough, and having less and less patience in rehearsals.

She spoke to the band director, who was in charge of musical direction of the show. He had noticed that she was taking on more responsibility than her predecessor.

"Why are you doing all of that?" he asked her. "That is the job of your stage manager, assistant director, stage crew—you don't do any of that."

"But they asked for my help."

"Of course. They're little baby birds taking their first steps out of the nest. Let them take risks."

She felt herself flinch from the idea that her baby birds might fall, naturally identifying with the mother hen. "How do I do that?" she asked.

He shrugged. "You just do it."

Mmmmmkay.

Julie realized that her "mother henning" was the problem. As a mother hen, she was putting not just the needs, but also the wishes, desires, and total comfort of her students ahead of her own work and sanity.

She wondered if "father cocking" was a thing.

Julie decided to invent it. She began responding to anyone's assumption that she would take on their respon-

*sibilities for them by either telling them that they could handle that task themselves or giving them a name of someone who might be able to help. After a few weeks of this, she compared notes with the band director, and he confirmed that her new approach was more like her predecessor's.*

*It was not a universal success. Students complained. Her administrators asked her why she wasn't taking charge of the play.*

*"I am taking charge," she said. "I'm doing everything my predecessor did, everything the director across town does. I'm asking the students to take initiative."*

*"Well, they say they don't feel that you're supporting them."*

*Why did the students feel differently about her as a director than their previous director?*

*"Human Giver Syndrome," Amelia suggested. "The expectations for women are different from men, even if no one says it out loud."*

*"So . . . what do I do?"*

*"Keep doing your job, being awesome at it, and eventually the people you work with get used to the fact that you're a person, an individual, a director. Their old expectations will be eroded by your competence."*

*Julie tried and it helped. Father cocking was smoothing her path through the gendered expectations of her job.*

*But again, it would turn out not to be enough.*

## The "Tall Tree" Fairness Test

We can imagine the advantages and disadvantages that shape our lives as similar to the natural environment that shapes a tree as it grows. A tree growing on an open, level field grows straight and tall, toward the sun; a tree that grows on a hillside will also grow toward the sun—which means it will grow at an angle. The steeper the hill, the sharper the angle of the tree, so if we transplant that tree to the level field, it's going to be a totally different shape from a tree native to that field. Both are adapted to the environment where they grew. We can infer the shape of the environment where a tree grew by looking at the shape of the tree.

White men grow on an open, level field. White women grow on far steeper and rougher terrain because the field wasn't made for them. Women of color grow not just on a hill, but on a cliffside over the ocean, battered by wind and waves. None of us chooses the landscape in which we're planted. If you find yourself on an ocean-battered cliff, your only choice is to grow there, or fall into the ocean. So if we transplant a survivor of the steep hill and cliff to the level field, natives of the field may look at that survivor and wonder why she has so much trouble trusting people, systems, and even her own bodily sensations. Why is this tree so bent and gnarled?

It's because that is what it took to survive in the place where she grew. A tree that's fought wind and gravity and erosion to grow strong and green on a steep cliff is going to look strange and out of place when moved to the level playing field. The gnarled, wind-blown tree from an oceanside cliff might not conform with our ideas of what a tree should look like, but it works well in the context where it grew. And that tall straight tree wouldn't stand a chance if it was transplanted to the cliffside.[19]

One kind of adversity: How many white parents do you know who explicitly teach their children to keep their hands in sight at all times and always say "Yes, sir" and "No, ma'am" if they are stopped by the police? That's just standard operating procedure for a lot of African American parents. Black parents in America grow their kids differently, because the landscape their kids are growing in requires it. The stark difference between how people of color are treated by police and how white people are treated results in white people thinking black people are ridiculous for being afraid of the police. We can't see the ocean, so when black people tell us, "We do this to avoid falling into the ocean," we don't understand. But just because we can't see it doesn't mean it's not there. How can we tell? By looking at the shape of the tree. Trees that grow at an angle grew on the side of a hill. People who are afraid of the police grew up in a world where the police are a threat.[20]

Just because the road looks flat doesn't mean it is. Just because you can't see the ocean doesn't mean it's not there. You can infer the landscape by looking at the shapes of the people who grew in those environments. Instead of wondering why they aren't thriving on the level playing field, imagine how the field can be changed to allow everyone to thrive.

---

### COMPASSION FATIGUE

The patriarchy (ugh) not only affects us directly, but also causes indirect harm to us as we care for others. When we experience stress on behalf of others, we may dismiss it as inconsequential or "irrational" and ignore it. Givers may spend years attending to the needs of others, while dismissing their own stress generated in response to witnessing those needs. The result is uncountable incomplete stress response cycles accumulating in our bodies. This accumulation leads to "compassion fatigue," and it's a primary cause of burnout among givers, including those who work in helping professions (many of which are dominated by women—teaching, social work, healthcare, etc). Signs of compassion fatigue include[21]

• checking out, emotionally—faking empathy when you know you're supposed to feel it, because you can't feel the real thing anymore;

• minimizing or dismissing suffering that isn't the most extreme—"It's not slavery/genocide/child rape/nuclear war, so quit complaining";

• feeling helpless, hopeless, or powerless, while also feeling personally responsible for doing more; and

• staying in a bad situation, whether a workplace or a relationship, out of a sense of grandiosity—"If I don't do it, no one will."

People who live through traumatic experiences are called survivors.

People who love and support people who live through traumatic experiences are co-survivors. They need all the support and care that a survivor needs. If they don't get it, they run the risk of burning out, dropping out, and tuning out. If we want to change the world, we need change agents to know how to receive care.

Fortunately the skills you'll learn in the last section of this book—social connection, rest, and befriending your inner critic—are evidence-based strategies for recovering from and preventing compassion fatigue.[22]

It would be great if the world could maybe stop telling us how broken and crazy we are, but we don't have to wait for the world to change in order to stop feeling this way. We can start right now. It's what the rest of this book is about.

The first step is knowing the game is rigged—seeing the way the rules are set up not just to treat some people unequally, but also to blind us to the unfairness of the rules.

The next steps are to apply the first three chapters of the book: (1) Complete the cycle, to deal with the stress itself. (2) Use planful problem-solving and positive reappraisal, to keep your Monitor satisfied. And (3) engage with your Something Larger, which will heal Human Giver Syndrome.

## 1. Complete the Cycle: Feels About the Patriarchy

As Gloria Steinem wrote, "The truth will set you free, but first it will piss you off." Seeing the rigged game isn't a neutral experience; you'll probably feel some feelings about it as you go through the world spotting the ways the game is rigged and the ways the world is lying to you about the ways the game is rigged. These feelings are uncomfortable, and when they get really intense it's tempting to ignore them and just stop playing. In other words: burnout. So let's not ignore them.

Rage is a big one. A lot of us are carrying around decades of incomplete stress response cycles because Human Giver Syndrome told us we had to be happy and calm and not make other people uncomfortable with our anger. Move, sing, scream, write, chop wood. Purge the rage. Complete the cycle.

Grief is another big one. We mourn for the loss of the life we might have had, the person we might have been, if we had been born into a world that believed women are 100 percent people and that men should be attentive to the needs of others. And it's complicated, too, because this lying, unfair world made you who you are, and a lot of who you are is pretty amazing, right? Not perfect, no one is perfect, but wow. *Wow.*

What do you do with the grief? You go through the tunnel. You allow it to move through you. Each time, your best self, the part that makes you go "Wow!"—even if you don't yet know who she is—will be with you as you grieve; she is the light at the end.

And there's despair. Despair is different from grief. It's the helpless, hopeless feeling we get when our Monitors give up on a goal, deciding it is unattainable.

Fortunately, science can help us with despair.

## 2. Unlearning Helplessness: Do a Thing

In those small, short-term experimental conditions, just telling the helpless human that the game is rigged was enough to make them feel better. But when learned helplessness has been induced over a lifetime of experience, you need to teach your nervous system that it's not helpless.

How?

You do something—and "something" is anything that isn't nothing. The patriarchy (ugh) is designed like the perfect shuttle-box experiment, frustrating and disappointing us over and over until we give up. But that research also demonstrated how helplessness can be unlearned.

Here's how they did it for dogs: After inducing learned helplessness, experimenters physically dragged the dogs over the barrier to the safe side of the shuttle box, over and over. By moving its body and consequently changing its situation, the experimenters led the dog to learn that its physical efforts could result in change.

Humans can unlearn helplessness the same way. In chapter 1, we learned that you don't have to deal with a stressor directly to deal with the stress itself. Helplessness works the same way. When you feel trapped, free yourself from *anything*, and it will teach your body that you are not helpless.

For instance, feeling helpless and hopeless after watching news about the state of international politics? Don't distract yourself or numb out; do a thing. Do yard work or gardening, to care for your small patch of the world. Take food to somebody who needs a little boost. Take your dog to the park. Show up at a Black Lives Matter march. You might even call your government representative. That's great. That's participation. You're not helpless. Your goal is not to stabilize the government—that's not your job (unless you happen to be a person whose job that is, in which case you still need to deal with the stress, as well as the stressor!)—your goal is to stabilize *you,* so that you can maintain a sense of efficacy, so that you can do the important stuff your family and your community need from you. As the saying goes, "Nobody can do everything, but everybody can do something." And "something" is anything that isn't nothing.

It's likely that you've received the message that when you're feeling overwhelmed with helplessness it's because you just can't be "rational," you're just overreacting, and the problem is your "mindset" or your weakness or just generally your *fault.* You should be able to do just as well as any man, and if you can't, the problem is you.

It's not true, and the people who say it is are gaslighting you. The truth is you learned helplessness from experiences of *being helpless.*

We unlearn helplessness by *doing a thing*—a thing that uses our body. Go for a walk. Scream into a pillow. Or, as Carrie Fisher put it, "Take your broken heart, make it into art." Reverse the effects of helplessness by creating a context where you can *do* a thing.

In the animated movie *Finding Nemo,* we get to know Dory the blue tang, a friendly fish who suffers from short-term memory loss. Famously voiced by Ellen DeGeneres, Dory advises her friends to "just keep swimming" when things are difficult. She even sings a song about it. In *Finding Dory,* we learn (spoiler) that it was her parents who taught her that even with her short-term memory loss, there was always a way to get through a difficulty. If you just keep swimming, you'll find your way. And when your brain wants to give up because there's no land in sight, you keep swimming, not because you're certain swimming will take you where you want to go, but to prove to yourself that you can still swim.

### 3. Smash

You're completing the cycle. You're *doing* things, using your body, to remind yourself that you are not helpless.

Step three: Smash the patriarchy. Smash it to pieces.

You smash it by making meaning—engaging with your Something Larger in ways that heal Human Giver Syndrome.

**SMASHIN'-SOME-PATRIARCHY WORKSHEET**

My Something Larger is: _____

_____

Something I do to engage with my Something Larger that also smashes some patriarchy is: _____

_____

_____

_____

I'll know I smashed some patriarchy when . . .
(soon, certain, positive, concrete, specific, and personal): _____

_____

A caveat: Don't smash with the goal of "ending the patriarchy." You are not going to see the end of gender inequality or racial inequality or any other inequality. You are going to see *progress,* just as you can see that progress has happened over the last hundred years. Instead, your goal—which, remember, should be soon, certain, positive, concrete, specific, and personal—can be something like "Buy all my friends' birthday presents from woman-owned stores." Or "In every meeting, invite women to speak first." Or "Give my boys a lesson each day in being a human giver." Or just "SMASH DAILY." Put a reminder in your calendar. Did you smash today?

> *Sophie was practicing explaining the unwinnable game to Emily.*
>
> *"Nobody would need this workshop if they could just spend an hour being me. People ask if my hair is real. My doctor tells me I'm too fat for him to take my pulse. Teenagers throw garbage at me from their car while I'm walking down the sidewalk . . ."*
>
> *"And yet you don't blow up the building," Emily said. "You're a frickin' superhero."*
>
> *"Yes," Sophie said emphatically. "Racism, sexism, sizeism, microaggressions, macroaggressions—this system is brutal, and there's no beating it. It's the Kobayashi Maru. None of us is getting out of this alive. But I win every time because I prove my character. Look how strong it made me. Look how smart it made me." She gestured down at herself. "Look how hot it made me."*
>
> *Emily nodded. "You are the new hotness."*
>
> *What Emily meant by that is the subject of the next chapter.*

Looking at the scale and scope of the rigging can be painful—scary and enraging and overwhelming. No wonder people hate the word "patriarchy." It's a word that exposes and names a source of pain so old and deep we've learned to ignore it or treat it as if it's how life should be. In general, "self-help"-type books try to help people feel good, empowered, in control of their lives, so they leave this chapter out. Acknowledging the large-scale social forces that surround you does not necessarily feel good, empowering, or like you're in control.

But it's also like looking at the climate. It's where you live. You can't escape it. And you can change it only in tiny, tiny increments. If you don't plan for it, you won't know when to plant and when to harvest. If you don't acknowledge it, you won't notice that it's changing, that your world is being cooked alive, and you won't be able to fix it.

And we're not done. There's another enemy, one you confront each and every day. It tells you it's your friend, when really it's trying to kill you slowly.

That's what the next chapter is about.

## tl;dr:

- The game is rigged. Women and girls—especially women and girls of color—are systematically excluded from government and other systems of power. It's called "patriarchy" (ugh).

- The patriarchy (ugh) says it doesn't exist. It says that if we struggle, it's our own fault for not being "good enough." Which is gaslighting.

- Human Giver Syndrome—the contagious belief that you have a moral obligation to give every drop of your humanity in support of others, no matter the cost to you—thrives in the patriarchy, the way mold thrives in damp basements.

- The solution? SMASH. (See worksheet. ☺)

# 5

# THE BIKINI INDUSTRIAL COMPLEX

*Julie was working hard to manage her stress. She didn't feel great, but she was staying afloat. Until she wasn't.*

*Her stomach had been "off" for a few days, or maybe weeks, but she didn't see anything wrong when she looked in the mirror, so she didn't think about it. She got away with ignoring it until she woke up in the middle of the night with cramps she couldn't ignore.*

*The family had moved—always an exhausting process—and she spent her first night in the new house alternately curled up in bed, lying on the bathroom floor, or sitting on the unfamiliar toilet while nothing happened but cold sweat, shivering, and minor but uncontrollable . . . um . . . leakage. When she googled her symptoms, the Internet told Julie to SEE A DOCTOR IMMEDIATELY.*

*Three hours later, she was being examined in the ER. They pressed on her belly while spasms and cramps caused more leakage. Julie was too uncomfortable to feel embarrassed, but the word* embarrassed *started repeating itself in her head while they asked questions about risk factors: poor diet, sedentary lifestyle, Crohn's disease, recent abdominal surgery, opioid use . . . no, no, no, no, no. High stress and change of schedule? Julie felt her body contract, her face went hot, and she started to cry. The new job, all the tension with her husband . . . Doesn't everyone go through these things? Could these ordinary things land her in the emergency room?*

*After an unnerving scan, they had her diagnosis. It included the word "impaction." The good news was it was isolated and therefore treatable with a quick, easy procedure that included the word "scoop." And her follow-up care included the words "bowel retraining."*

*Now she felt embarrassed. Yeah, having a poop-related ER visit doesn't feel super-dignified, but it was worse than that. It was as though she had failed, as though her body was substandard because it seemed to have overreacted to the stress of her normal, average life.*

*"No, it's not a disproportionate response," Amelia told her over the phone the next day. "You may not have been aware of how bad it was, but your body was. Believe it when it tells you things."*

*"That sounds . . . I mean"—Julie hedged—"My body knows things? It tells me things? Come on, what actually happens?"*

*"Your body holds on to stress," Amelia explained unhelpfully.*

*"Well, why can't it handle my perfectly normal amount of stress?"*

*"Perfectly normal? You're changing jobs, moving houses, and maybe getting divorced—that's facing three*

*of the worst stressors known to the industrialized West all at once. What exactly are you expecting from your body?"*

*It turned out Julie's expectations for her body and what it was supposed to be were totally wrong. She thought she could measure her wellness by the appearance of her body. Of course she did; that's what we're all taught to do.*

*This chapter is about how Julie got it so wrong, and what she had to learn to get it right.*

On the day a girl is born, she may be lucky enough to have people around her who instantly welcome every roll on her body, every wrinkle on her fingers, every blotch on her skin, and each and every hair, no matter where it is, on her brand-new little body. Her little body is full of needs—needs for food, sleep, diaper changes, being held. The adults are there to listen to the distress signals that her body sends out, and when we're lucky, they willingly meet those needs, no matter how sleep-deprived, busy, or desperate they feel.

Most of us are met, at our birth, with an enveloping, protective love that holds and cherishes every inch of our bodies. In that moment and in that love, we are flawless. Beautiful.

And then.

And then we are infected with Human Giver Syndrome, which pushes girl babies to grow into human givers—pretty, happy, calm, generous, and attentive to the needs of others—while it pushes boy babies to be ambitious, competitive, strong, and infallible.

Picture that girl on the day of her birth, perfect and helpless and full of life, maybe held against the skin of a loving parent.

She's beautiful, right? She's perfect.

And she's you.

Here is the secret Human Giver Syndrome doesn't want you to know: Nothing has changed. No matter what has happened to that body of yours between the day you were born, beautiful and perfect, and the day you read this, your body is still beautiful and perfect. And it is still full of needs.

And yet by the age of six, about half of girls are worried about being "too fat."[1] By age eleven, it's up to two-thirds, and by full adolescence almost all girls will have engaged in some kind of "weight control" behavior.[2] One recent study of more than 4,500 adolescents found that nearly all of them (92 percent) engaged in some kind of weight-control behavior, and almost half (44 percent) of girls engaged in unhealthy weight-control behaviors.[3]

It hasn't always been like this, and it isn't like this everywhere; it happens because our culture makes it happen. In 1994, there was no television on the island of Fiji; there were also no eating disorders. British and American television were brought to the island in 1995. By 1998, 29 percent of the girls had developed severe eating disorder symptoms. Thirteen percent developed these symptoms *within one month* of the introduction of television.[4]

But in a sense, it has always been like this, and it is like this everywhere. Every culture has an "aspirational beauty ideal" that women are encouraged to strive for. Our own grandmother told us stories from the 1930s, when her family was so poor they lived in a house their father had built from scraps; they were lucky to have a toilet, but it was plumbed into the middle of the house, with no privacy. She and her sisters were thin; in fact, they had grown up on the edge of starvation. Still, in high school the three girls scraped together money to buy "diet aids," which were supposed to last them a month. The "aids" turned out to be candy (because sugar was supposed to be an appetite suppressant) and they ate the whole box in one afternoon.

And it isn't just white people or Western culture. Taiwanese American Lynn Chen, founder of thickdumplingskin.com, describes explicit expectations from her Taiwanese parents "to eat large quantities of food but remain skinny," which shaped her problematic relationship with food and her body.[5]

*And* it doesn't have to be thinness. The Jamaican "ideal woman" has lots of curves, and girls have been known to take "chicken pills"—medication to fatten poultry—in order to obtain those curves. But the pills contain arsenic.[6]

Everywhere, there is a beauty ideal, and always, there are those willing to risk their health to attain it. Far from hearing the distress signals our body is sending, its desperate cries for food, sleep, being held, and, in Julie's case, bowel movements, we relate to our bodies only in terms of its appearance.

But imagine what it would be like to live in a culture where that feeling we had on the day we were born stayed the same all through our childhood and into adolescence, a culture that didn't constantly reinforce the idea that a girl's or woman's body is supposed to be one specific shape and size, and if it's not she must, at all costs, try to *make* it that shape and size. What if the shape we grew into was just accepted as the natural shape of our bodies, as lovable each new day as it was on the day we were born? What if the body we aged into—those of us lucky enough to grow old—was as beautiful in our own eyes, when we looked in the mirror, as worthy of love and protection, as the body we had on the day we were born? What if the shape of our bodies was peripheral to our relationship with our bodies, and we could pay compassionate attention to our body's needs without assessing whether it "deserves" food or love?

What if?

This is the chapter where we teach you how to love your body.

## The Bikini Industrial Complex

This is our name for the hundred-billion-dollar cluster of businesses that profit by setting an unachievable "aspirational ideal" for us, convincing us that we both can and should—indeed we *must*—conform with the ideal, and then selling us ineffective but plausible strategies for achieving that ideal.[7] It's like old cat pee in the carpet, powerful and pervasive and it makes you uncomfortable every day—but it's invisible and no one can remember a time when it didn't smell. Let's spend a few paragraphs shining a black light on it, so you can know where the smell is coming from.

You already know that everything in the media is there to sell you thinness—the shellacked abs in advertisements for exercise equipment, the ONE WEIRD TRICK TO LOSE BELLY FAT clickbait when all you wanted was a weather forecast, and princesses played by "flawless" thin women on TV. The Bikini Industrial Complex, or BIC, has successfully created a culture of immense pressure to conform to an ideal that is literally unobtainable by almost everyone and yet is framed not just as the most beautiful, but the healthiest and most virtuous.

But it's not just magazine covers and other fictions that get it wrong. Even your high school health class had it wrong. Your doctor had it wrong, because her medical textbooks had it wrong, because the federal government had it wrong. Like "Big Oil" and "Big Tobacco," "Big Bikini" has lobbied government agencies to make sure their products have the support of Congress. The body mass index (BMI) chart and its labels—underweight, overweight, obese, etc.—were created by a panel of nine individuals, seven of whom were "employed by weight-loss clinics and thus have an economic interest in encouraging use of their facilities."[8]

You've been lied to about the relationship between weight and health so that you will perpetually try to change your weight.

But listen: It can be healthier to be seventy or more pounds over your medically defined "healthy weight" than just five pounds under it. A 2016 meta-analysis published in *The Lancet* examined 189 studies, encompassing nearly four million people who never smoked and had no diagnosed medical issues. It found that people labeled "obese" by the Centers for Disease Control and Prevention (CDC) have *lower health risk* than those the CDC categorized as "underweight." The study also found that being "overweight" according to the CDC is *lower risk* than being at the low end of the "healthy" range, as defined by the U.S. federal government and the World Health Organization (WHO). [9]

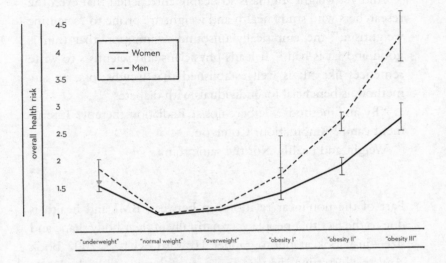

Another meta-analysis even found that people in the BMI category labeled "overweight" may live longer than people in any other category, and the highest predictable mortality rate might be among those labeled "underweight."[10]

"What?" you ask, in disbelief.

"Exactly!" we respond.

*"What?"* you ask again.

"I know!" we reply. "It's bananas!"

Even research that describes itself as contradicting these meta-analyses and confirming that "overweight" is bad concedes, "We do not yet have convincing data from *randomized controlled trials* in humans that methods used for promoting weight loss among obese persons prolong life [emphasis original]."[11] Translation: Even if you lose weight by buying whatever advice they're selling (and there's no scientific reason to believe you will), don't expect to live longer. Taking it even further, the newest research is suggesting doctors warn middle-aged and older patients *against* losing weight, because the increasingly well-established dangers of fluctuations in weight outweigh any risk associated with a high but stable weight.[12]

And yet weight stigma is so deeply entrenched that even the researchers who study health and weight are prone to "scientific weightism," the empirically unsound assumption that thin is good and fat is bad.[13] It leads physicians and scientists to write sentences like "It is well established that weight loss, by any method, is beneficial for individuals with diabetes."[14]

"By any method"? Tuberculosis? Radiation therapy? Internment camp? Amputation? Come on.

Weight and health. Not the same thing.

Part of the nonlinear relationship between BMI and health is due to the fact that people vary naturally in their body shape and size—just look at photographer Howard Schatz's 2002 book *Athlete,* illustrating the vast and beautiful range of body shapes and sizes of Olympic athletes.[15] Every one of those people, from the tiniest gymnast to the biggest weight lifter, is at the absolute peak of their sport. Health comes in every shape and size; some people are healthiest at a lower BMI and some are healthiest at a higher BMI.

But part of this is because the BMI is *nonsense* as a measure of personal health. It's literally just a ratio of height to weight, which is why a doctor told one of Emily's students—an internationally competitive figure skater, i.e., a professional athlete—that she was "overweight," even though she was so low-body-fat that she was skipping periods. She had so much muscle and such dense bones that she weighed as much as a man her height. And again, even studies that assume body fat is dangerous agree that BMI misclassifies as "healthy" *half* of people who are "normal or just overweight," but who are nevertheless at risk for all the health issues associated with obesity.[16] People of any size can be healthy or sick; you can't tell by looking at them.

Does the BMI chart mention that this codification of "health" relies more on bias than on science?[17] Nope. It just labels people as "unhealthy," ignores the science, and gives physicians and insurance companies government sanctioning to collect fees for treatment of this "disease."[18]

And we all believe it, because our culture has primed us to judge fat people as lazy and selfish.

But it's even bigger than that. Here's how deep it goes:

Amelia conducts a children's choir, and she has to teach her kids to breathe. At ten, eight, even six years old, they already believe that bellies are supposed to be flat and hard, and so they hold their stomachs in. You can't breathe deeply, all the way, without relaxing your abdomen, and you can't sing if you can't breathe. So Amelia has to teach children to breathe. Amelia's young singers show that the BIC doesn't just teach us to ignore our needs for food and love; it doesn't even want us to *breathe*. Not all the way.

Relax your belly. It's supposed to be round. The Bikini Industrial Complex has been gaslighting you.

We're not saying the people or companies that constitute the Bikini Industrial Complex are out to get you. Frankly, we don't think they're smart enough to have created this screwed-up system on purpose. But we're far from the first to recognize there's money to be made by establishing and enforcing impossible standards by which we're told to measure ourselves.

## Stigma Is the Health Hazard

What is the cost of the Bikini Industrial Complex's success?

There is, of course, the financial cost: the aforementioned hundred-billion-dollar global industry thrives on our body dissatisfaction, and the less effective it is at making our bodies "fit," the more money it makes, as we try product after product, trend after trend.

And there is opportunity cost: With the time and money we spend on worrying about the shape of our bodies and attempting to make them "fit," what else might we accomplish? Along with that comes "self-regulatory fatigue"; if you're using up decision-making and attention-focusing cognitive resources on choices about food, clothes, exercise, makeup, body hair, "toxins," and fretting about your body's failures, what are you too exhausted to care about, that you would otherwise prioritize?

There's also the chronic, low-level stress—like the rats with tilted cages and flashing lights—of navigating an environment filled with images of the ideal and people who believe in it. Even if you don't buy in, they'll be there to say, "How nice for you that you don't care," or "No, don't give up on yourself!" or "Aren't you worried about your health? What about your (my) insurance premiums?" What they're really saying is, "How dare you? If I have to follow the rules, then so do you. *Get back in line.*" As body activist Jes Baker says, "When a fat chick who *hasn't* done the work, who *hasn't* tried to fix her body, who *doesn't* have any interest in the gospel we so zealously believe in, *stands up and says:* I'M HAPPY! . . . we freak the fuck out. Because: that bitch just broke the rules. She just cut in front of us in line. She just unwittingly ripped us off. And she essentially made our lifetime of work totally meaningless."[19]

That "freak-out" leads to another cost: the discrimination. People of size are paid less at work, experience more bullying at school—not just from other kids, but from *teachers*—and have their symptoms dismissed or ignored by doctors, and thus go longer without appropriate diagnosis and treatment when they have actual medical problems.[20]

Then there is the cost in human health and life: Dieting—especially "yo-yo dieting," repeatedly gaining and losing weight—ultimately causes changes in brain functioning that increase insulin and leptin resistance (causing weight gain, which leads to dieting, and so on), which leads to actual disease. And eating disorders have the highest mortality of any mental illness—

higher even than depression—killing 250,000 people a year.[21] The thin ideal makes us sick. And it kills some of us.

And although a rising proportion of men struggle with body dysmorphia, and the cultural pressures around men's bodies are intensifying ("dad bod" notwithstanding), this remains a distinctly gendered issue.[22] It is women's time, money, mental energy, opportunity, health, and lives that are being drained away in the endless pursuit of a "better" body, and it starts as soon as we "gender" a child's toys. Very young girls' exposure to dolls with unrealistic body types increases their desire to be thin.[23] This despite the fact that the *Lancet* meta-analysis found that the health risk associated with low or high BMI was "far greater"— quoting the researchers—for men than for women. And yet who gets more flak from their culture and even, yes, from their doctors about their weight? Women, of course—twice as much as men.[24] Why? Because we're the "human givers"; we're the ones with a moral obligation to be pretty—that is, to conform to the aspirational ideal.

It gets worse. The body ideal is built into the physical infrastructure of society, from the size and shape of airplane seats to the weight-bearing capacity of medical tables. One friend of ours couldn't get a mammogram because the machine at the doctor's office didn't hold over 250 pounds—outrageously inexcusable, when 5 to 10 percent of American women over the age of forty weigh more than 250 pounds.[25]

This grotesque discrimination means that it *is* dangerous to be a fat person in the world—not because of the fat, but because of the daily discrimination, exclusion, and stigmatization.

Reasonable people may disagree about the specific relationship between weight and health. But there is no reasonable case to be made, no evidence at all, that stigma is anything but actively harmful. Which is why . . .

## It Would Be Nice to Be Thin

Owen Elliot, daughter of Cass Elliot of the band the Mamas and the Papas, has said of her mother, "She accepted who she was, a sexy woman who was never short of boyfriends, but I think if she could have been thinner, she would have. I'm overweight right now and I'm still beautiful. But God, it would be nice to be thin and I think that's where she was at, too."[26]

That fundamental ambivalence between accepting your body and changing your body is both common and rational. Despite the accumulating evidence that people of different shapes and sizes can be healthy, the stigma around body shape pervades every domain of our lives, and the prejudice, bias, false beliefs, and stigma against fat and fat people can literally kill you.[27] And this form of discrimination is not just legal but normalized, rationalized, by the incorrect idea that fat is a disease.

So yes indeed, it would be nice to be thin, because it would privilege us with the gift of being treated like actual people, no matter what. Thin privilege is as real as privilege associated with race, gender, and class. Women of color would face less adversity if they were white. Trans folks would face less adversity if they were cisgender. People on the autism spectrum would face less adversity if they were neurotypical. And, yes, fat people would face less adversity if they were thin. And none of those folks chose to be who they are. They can only choose to embrace who they are and try to tolerate living in a world that doesn't tolerate them.

Living in a body that is outside the "norm" can be a hassle when you're clothes shopping, frustrating when you're navigating public transportation, and exhausting when you're just trying to buy groceries without people offering their opinions—silently or otherwise. It is experienced as another "chronic stressor," like the rats who come home to find water poured all over their nests. And that stress accumulates.

The urge to conform is perfectly rational. And the BIC lies to you, tells you you *could* conform if you worked harder, had more discipline, on and on, bullshitbullshit, and the stress works its way from the outside to the inside. Even people who conform, more or less, to the aspirational ideal experience this stress. When they can't credibly be told they have to be thinner, thin people are told they should "sculpt" or "tone" their abs or arms or butt or thighs. And everyone, regardless of size, is supposed to fret over food choices and exercise and clothes that make you "look fat" in an effort to fit the precisely molded aspirational ideal. We've been taught that our bodies reflect our morality and indeed our very worth as human beings. Fat people are viewed as "lazy, glutinous [*sic*], greedy, immoral, uncontrolled, stupid, ugly, lacking in will power, primitive."[28] Thin people, by contrast, are self-controlled and nice and clean and smart. The stakes for conforming feel excruciatingly high.

People who tell you they're worried about your fat may say—they may even *believe*—they're worried about your health. But since fat isn't a disease, what they're really worried about is your social life. Being accepted by your culture. It would be nice to be thin.

---

### WHY THINNESS?

As Naomi Wolf puts it, "A culture fixated on female thinness is not an obsession about female beauty, but an obsession about female obedience." Thin bodies are the bodies of women who behave themselves.

Like so many toxic norms of the twenty-first century, the thin ideal is a by-product of the Industrial Revolution. Before that, a softer, rounder, plumper female was the beauty standard, because it was only the rich women who could afford the luxurious food and freedom from manual labor that allowed them to accumulate the abundant curves of the women in Rubens's paintings. But in the nineteenth century, with the rise of the middle class, it became fashionable for a man to be able to afford a wife who was too weak to work. It was a status symbol, an advertisement of wealth, for a man to have a wife who not only didn't but *couldn't* contribute to the household income. "Delicate" and "fragile" became feminine virtues.

This is in contradiction of everything evolution would have a woman be: robust, strong, able healthfully to conceive, gestate, birth, breastfeed, and carry multiple offspring.

So that, friends, is where the thin ideal originates—in the basic assumption that a woman is a man's property, his status symbol. Because: patriarchy. (Ugh.)

*Sophie has two sets of clothes—three if you count the Uhura cosplay. She has a work wardrobe, full of the kinds of things people expect a professional to wear, which she considers just as much a costume as the Uhura dress. And she has the leggings and screen-printed T-shirts that say things like "Joss Is My Master Now" and "What Would Geordi Do?"*

*So when the academic department for which she was consulting invited her out to dinner at the start of her gig, we went shopping with her.*

*Not many women make it to adulthood with as solid a sense of their own beauty as Sophie. She is a confident, body-positive woman of size. But then she has to go out in the world and try on dresses. This time she went to a fancy-pants department store, with valet parking and complimentary glasses of sparkling water. She chose a few things and went to try them on. She showed us a few op-*

tions, including one truly outstandingly hot one, then went to try on the next dress.

Which is when we overheard two other women just outside the dressing room. They were talking in hushed voices, but still plainly audible.

The first lady said, "It's like she doesn't even care! I'm sorry, I get up at five-thirty every morning and sweat my butt off on the treadmill. If she's too lazy or doesn't even respect herself enough to—" and at that point Emily's ears filled with the white noise of rageful blood pounding in her head.

Through the roar, she heard the other lady say, "I'm just genuinely worried about her health, you know? Like, she's a walking heart attack!"

"And now our taxes are subsidizing her slow death by Twinkies! Hashtag thanks, Obama!"

Tittering laughter.

We looked at each other. Emily looked at the door of Sophie's dressing room. Amelia went over to the ladies, because she's the one who goes over to people.

"We can hear you," she said.

They looked at her, uncomprehending.

"That's our friend you're talking about," Amelia said, and the penny dropped. They stammered and looked abashed, but also unimpressed—Amelia is herself not thin, which makes her lazy and a walking heart attack, too, so why would they care about her opinion? Still, Amelia continued on an angry tirade, explaining Health at Every Size and that size discrimination is the last haven of sanctioned prejudice, and Emily just stood there, struggling to believe this kind of thing actually happens.

As Amelia's voice was starting to get to making-a-scene volume, Sophie came out of the dressing room wearing her own clothes, with the totally hot dress slung over one arm.

*"Should we leave?" Emily asked her.*

*"Oh, we're leaving," Sophie said, loud enough for the ladies to hear, then winked at Emily. "But first I'm buying this hot dress."*

*Three slow deep breaths later, Sophie was signing the sales slip with us right behind her, and the uncomfortable ladies in a clutch by the dressing room.*

*Emily said, "This is going to be a really funny story, a few months from now."*

*"It's already funny," Sophie said.*

*And she wore that totally hot dress to the dinner, where she would meet the love of her life.*

## Your New "Weight Loss Goal"

"Just give me a number! What should I *weigh*????" you ask.

Wouldn't it be great if it were that simple?

On top of all the individual variability we discussed, another major reason why it's not that simple is something called "defended weight." Just as some people are night owls and others are larks and our body rhythms change across our life-span, so some people are big and others are small, and our bodies change across our life-span. The basic shape and size of your adult body has what neuroscientist Sandra Aamodt calls a "defended weight" that it will protect. Eat a little extra one day, your appetite will be smaller the next day. Starve yourself for three months to fit the bridesmaid dress your best friend got you . . . then eat like you've been starving for three months, until your body returns to its defended weight. Defended weight tends to go up as we age and almost never goes down. Only a very small fraction of the population can lose weight and sustain that weight loss through diet and exercise, establishing a new defended weight.[29]

How frustrating is this information? Is part of you still certain there's a different weight you ought to be, and could be if only you had the discipline?

Back in chapter 2, we talked about "when to quit." We suggested you make a grid—short- and long-term benefits of keeping this goal, and short- and long-term benefits of letting go of this goal. Try that with whatever your current body goal is.

Or you can listen to your inner voice, which has probably been begging for mercy for years.

You might choose to keep trying to change your body. It's your body and your decision. At least now you can adjust your expectations about just how difficult and long the effort will be.

You might choose to let go of trying to conform to the culturally constructed aspirational beauty ideal—again, your body, your choice. Then comes the hard part. An hour later, the BIC will be arguing with you, blaming and judging you, pressuring you to get back in line.

You're going to have to meet the BIC in daily combat, for your individual and our collective well-being. So let's look at four real-life strategies for making it through the fray.

## Strategy 1: Mess Acceptance

Multiple approaches to combating the BIC have been established over the last few decades, and a strong and growing foundation of research shows they're effective at improving health, preventing eating disorders, and reducing the mood and anxiety problems that accompany body self-criticism. Though the approaches vary, they also have a lot in common: they all encourage you to (1) practice body acceptance, (2) embrace body diversity, and (3) listen to your body.

Those things are good for you.[30] You should definitely try them.

But neither of us has ever met any woman whose relationship

with her body was not in some way equivocal—and no wonder. It's difficult to maintain body acceptance in the midst of the BIC, where you're surrounded by images of the ideal and by loved ones who say, "But you're going to lose the weight, right?"

Ambivalence is normal. So rather than aiming for "body acceptance," practice "mess acceptance." Turn toward the mess of noisy, contradictory thoughts and feelings with kindness and compassion. You know what's true now—your body size doesn't dictate your health; the Bikini Industrial Complex doesn't care about your health; it's all just patriarchy and capitalism and stuff—but knowing what's true doesn't magically cure it. Knowledge may be half the battle, but only half.

When you engage in physical activity, you know it's good for you, because: completing the cycle and also: doing a thing. You also know that most people probably assume you're trying to "lose weight" or "get in shape," and part of you might still actively want to change the shape of your body. That's all perfectly normal. Move your body anyway—because it really is good for you—and smile benevolently at the mess. Some days it will be messy as hell, other days it will be calm and clear, and every day is just part of the intensely body-neurotic world you happen to live in.

## Strategy 2: You Are the New Hotness

All the evidence-based models also include some redefinition of "beauty." When we reconstruct our own standard of beauty with a definition that comes from our own hearts and includes our bodies as they are right now, we can turn toward our bodies with kindness and compassion.

Easier said than done.

Amelia is vain about pictures of her conducting, in which she inevitably has her mouth wide open and her hair is a sweaty wreck. Emily watches herself on TV and worries that her chin is too pointy because one time, years ago, somebody said it was.

Neither of us has ever had the skinny proportions of a model, and we watched our mom (who was model-thin before she gestated two seven-pound babies at the same time) look at her reflection in dressing room mirrors and cry at what she saw there. What she saw there is very much like what we see in our own reflections now.

Which is why we play the "New Hotness" game, a strategy for teaching ourselves to let go of body self-criticism and shift to self-kindness.

One day, Amelia was in a dressing room of a very fancy boutique, trying on gowns for a performance she had coming up. Attire for women conductors is hard to find: solid black with long sleeves, formal, professional, yet not frumpy is an unlikely combination. Finding all of this in her size, right on the boundary between "straight" sizes and "plus" sizes, is even more difficult. So there she was at the fancy store, and she tried on a dress that looked so amazingly good that she texted Emily a dress selfie, with a caption paraphrasing Will Smith in *Men in Black II:* I AM THE NEW HOTNESS.

And now "new hotness" is our texting shorthand for looking fabulous without reference to the socially constructed ideal.

We recommend it. It's fun.

Maybe you don't look like you used to, or like you used to imagine you should; but how you look today is the *new* hotness. Even better than the old hotness.

Wearing your new leggings today? You are the new hotness.

Hair longer or shorter, or a different color or style? New hotness.

Saggy belly skin from that baby you birthed? New hotness.

Gained twenty pounds while finishing school? New hotness.

Skin gets new wrinkles because you lived another year? New hotness.

Scar tissue following knee replacement surgery? New hotness.

Amputation following combat injury? New hotness.

Mastectomy following breast cancer? New hotness.

The point is, *you* define and redefine your body's worth, on your own terms. Again and again, you turn toward your body with kindness and compassion.

It's not necessary to turn toward your body with love and affection—love and affection are frosting on the cake of body acceptance, and if they work for you, go for it.[31] All your body requires of you is that you turn toward it with kindness and compassion, with nonjudgment and plain-vanilla acceptance of all your contradictory emotions, beliefs, and longings.

We're not saying that "beautiful" is what your body *should* be; we're saying beautiful is what your body already is.

## Strategy 3: Everybody Is the New Hotness

Writer, comedian, and fat-positive activist Lindy West discovered her new hotness from exposure to positive images of fat bodies, and recommends that other women "look at pictures of fat women on the Internet until they don't make you uncomfortable anymore." She says Leonard Nimoy's *The Full Body Project* "came to me like a gift." She had never seen fat bodies like hers "presented without scorn . . . honored instead of lampooned . . . displayed as objects of beauty instead of punch lines." And she asked herself, "What if I could just decide I was valuable and it would be true?" And she felt it reshaping her brain. She later discovered the research that demonstrates that mere exposure to certain body types makes people prefer those body types.

At the end of some of her talks, Emily leads what she calls "The Beautiful Activity." She has a set of fifty PowerPoint slides, each with the image of someone who goes by the pronoun "she," along with the words "She is so beautiful." One at a time, going around the room, participants look at the image they're presented with and say out loud, "She is so beautiful." Then the next slide comes up and the next person says, "She is so beautiful." And the next slide, and the next person. There are women of every skin tone and hair texture, women with or without arm-pit hair, women in wheelchairs or with prosthetic limbs, women with single or double mastectomies, transgender women, an-drogynous women, women in burkas, women of every size, women of every age from their teens to their nineties.

The original idea of the exercise was that everyone in the room would see someone who looks like herself, and hear some-one declare that person beautiful. But it turned out, even more powerful was the feeling of dissonance participants experience, seeing a body that they've been taught to perceive with aversion and being challenged to try on the idea that that body is beauti-ful. Emily has led this activity with everyone from college stu-dents to seasoned therapists to medical providers, and the response is the same: tears and an astonished awareness of how uncomfortable it is, at first, to view non-"ideal" bodies without judgment . . . and of how quickly it becomes a source of joy.

You will finish this chapter and go out into the world and notice the diversity of bodies around you . . . and you will still have these reflexive, judgmental thoughts about the people who don't conform to the aspirational ideal, or those envious, con-temptuous thoughts about the people who do, or those self-critical, scolding thoughts about the ways the world tells you you fall short. It will happen any time you're out in public—on a train or a bus, standing in line at the checkout counter, at a party, at a work meeting, in a classroom. You'll notice other people's bodies, and you'll have an emotional reaction to them. And then you might even have emotional reactions to your emotional reactions—"Darn it, I shouldn't think that!"

That's all part of the mess. Change happens gradually. Your brain has been soaking in the BIC for decades; and any time you step outside your door, you're back in it; any time you turn on a television, you're back in it; any time you put clothes on or take clothes off, you're back in it. Just notice it, as you'd notice a fleck of dust floating through the air. Utterly neutral. No need to do anything about it. Smile kindly at the mess. And know what's true: Everyone is the new hotness. You are the new hotness. So is she. So are they. So are we.

## Strategy 4: "Hi Body, What Do You Need?"

Finally, turn your attention away from the mirror and other people's bodies, and notice what it feels like inside your body. Greet your internal sensations with the same kindness and compassion you practiced when you thought about the shape of your body.

When an infant squirms or cries because something about her body feels uncomfortable, the grown-ups have to figure out what the issue is, and we teach the infant what her body's sensations mean.[32] We coo, "Hi, honey, what's wrong? What do you need? Are you hungry? Tired? Lonely? Oh, you're hungry, huh?"

And the baby learns that that specific uncomfortable sensation means "hungry." Another uncomfortable sensation means "wet." A different uncomfortable sensation is "lonely."

But even as she grows more familiar with her body's internal sensations, she absorbs contradictory cultural messages about how she should feel about her body. The adults say things like "Look at that cute fat belly! I'm gonna zerbert that belly!" about her belly, and they also say, "Ugh, look at this fat belly, I'm so gross," about their own belly.

Even before she can read or speak, she watches commercials and sees the magazine covers at the grocery store, and though she may never talk about it with any of the people in her life, she is absorbing the idea that her body is not already beautiful and that if she doesn't make it beautiful, she doesn't automatically deserve food or love or rest or health. And as a budding "human giver," she learns that her body isn't for her, it's for other people. Other people's pleasure, other people's desire, other people's acceptance or rejection.

Many of us have grown into world-class ignorers of our own

needs, just as we were taught to be. We don't even notice that we're ignoring our needs. Our bodies are sending us all kinds of signals, but we live from the neck up, only attending to the noise in our heads and shutting out the noise coming from the other 95 percent of our internal experience.

Imagine that your body is the body of someone who needs your care, like an infant. It feels weird and wrong to a lot of us at first, but give it a try. Instead of just *looking* at your body to evaluate her well-being (we know that you can't tell anything about a person's health by the shape or size of their body), turn to her and ask her how she feels: "What's wrong, honey? Are you hungry? Thirsty? Tired? Lonely?" She can definitely tell you, if you listen. You might have to stop what you're doing, take a slow breath, focus on the sensation of your weight on the floor or the chair, and actually ask out loud, "What do you need?" You may receive the answer as an instantaneous knowing, or as a physical sensation you need to interpret, or as words in your mind. But she will give you an answer.

Though the details of her needs change as you grow—How much sleep, and when? Loving attention from whom? What kind of food?—the fundamentals do not. Your body needs to breathe and to sleep. She needs food. She needs love. She dies without them. And there is nothing she has to do, no shape or size she has to be, before she "deserves" food and love and sleep. It's not her fault if she's sick or injured. She's still the astonishing creature she was on the day she was born, a source of joy for those who care about her. She's yours.

She's you.

*Julie had literally never thought about what her body felt like. She paid attention to what it looked like, and, like most of us, spent a lot of time and effort on making it look thin enough; she followed diets she read about, did work-outs suggested by fitness gurus, and avoided clothes with horizontal stripes.*

*But her prescribed bowel retraining forced her to pay attention to how her body felt instead of how it looked.*

*A lot of body-positive talk emphasizes loving your body for "what it does" rather than how it looks, which is great as far as it goes. But it's not so helpful for Julie or anyone living with chronic pain or illness. Even though her body looked a lot like she thought healthy bodies were supposed to look, it had failed pretty catastrophically to do what bodies were supposed to do.*

*So she had to start from scratch, rebuilding her relationship with her body according to rules set by her body. There were guidelines to follow about food, but instead of a list of foods she could and couldn't eat, she was told to pay attention to how various foods felt in her body. It turned out what made her body feel good was radically different from any diet she had followed. There were instructions for way more sleep and exercise than she had ever had before, and how the hell was she going to be good to her body and also live her actual life?*

*She realized this question—this tradeoff between her body's needs and her life—was what put her in the hospital in the first place.*

*In order to make this work, she would need help. A lot of help.*

Bodies are imperfect, and sometimes they let us down. They are susceptible to disease and breakage and entropy. Our bodies can disappoint us, and the world can punish us when our bodies aren't what they "should" be. So we are not suggesting that you "love your body," like that's an easy fix. We're suggesting you be patient with your body and with your feelings about your body.

Your body is not the enemy. The real enemy is out there—the Bikini Industrial Complex. It is trying sneakily to convince you that you are the problem, that your body is the enemy, that your body is inadequate, which makes you a failure.

This stuff is difficult and messy. After you finish this chapter, you are going to have dinner with friends and hear them talking about calories and fat and whether or not they "deserve" to eat dessert or how nice it must be for you "not to care what you eat." You are going to hear family members criticize themselves or others for the way they've "let themselves go." You're going to want to explain to them that people don't need to *earn* the pleasure of delicious food, that de-prioritizing conformation with the culturally constructed ideal is not failure, and that "fat" doesn't mean "unhealthy." Sometimes you'll say these things; sometimes you won't. Sometimes you won't want the argument. Both choices are okay; it's all just part of the mess.

We'll conclude this chapter with this example of our own mess.

At the same time that Emily was working on this chapter, she was also—oh, God—losing weight, in preparation for a large professional event, to which she had been invited as a keynote speaker. She knows from the research and from experience that she is perceived differently depending on her weight, and she wanted to be perceived in the thin way. So one Friday morning, she spent three hours writing about body acceptance, and then she went upstairs and, because it was Friday, she weighed herself.

Then she called Amelia and said, "This is so screwed up! On the one hand, I really will be taken more seriously as a professional and an expert if I conform more closely to the aspirational ideal. On the other hand, my efforts to conform to that ideal are in opposition to the very message about which I have been invited to speak, as an expert."

"Yep, it's a mess," Amelia agreed. "But it's also the new hotness."

We started, back in Part I, with the resources we carry with us into this battle, the resources that stop the bleeding. Here in

Part II, we've described the tricky nature of this enemy, who tries to convince us it is our ally even as it shanks us between our ribs. In Part III we'll describe, in concrete, specific detail, how to win. We'll describe what that daily battle for just a little more ground, just a little more peace, looks and feels like. And we'll tell you about the personal, practical, and everyday things you can do to grow mighty.

### tl;dr:

- The "Bikini Industrial Complex" is a hundred-billion-dollar industry that tries to convince us that our bodies are the enemy, when, in reality, the Bikini Industrial Complex is itself the enemy.

- Bias against people of size can be more dangerous to our health than the actual size of our bodies. And many of the things we do to try to change our bodies make our health *worse*.

- It is normal—nearly universal—to feel ambivalent about your body, wanting to accept and love your body as it is and, at the same time, wanting to change it to conform to the culturally constructed aspirational ideal.

- Solutions: Embrace the mess. See yourself as "the new hotness." Practice seeing *everyone* as "the new hotness." And tune in to your body's needs.

# PART III

# Wax On, Wax Off

# 6

# CONNECT

*Sophie refers to herself as a Grown-Ass Woman. She supports herself financially, lives alone, and is your textbook independent female. She takes pride in knowing she can do things for herself, that she doesn't need anyone. She has family and friends for company, and she enjoys the romantic thrill of dating, but she doesn't share her life with anyone long-term. She wasn't all that interested in a relationship.*

*Until Bernard.*

*She met him while she was consulting at a big, famous technical university, helping them design more inclusive STEM programs. At the department dinner, she approached one of the few empty chairs, next to a man with frizzy hair.*

*"Is this seat taken?" she asked.*

*He looked up at her, clearly distracted by whatever he had been reading, and their eyes locked and she had no idea what he said. His eyes were sparkly and his expression was warm and welcoming. He had freckles. She felt like the earth had shifted out from under her; without any warning, she was suddenly standing in a new place.*

*He gestured to the empty seat, so she sat. Her stomach was suddenly full of butterflies.*

*"I'm Bernard," the guy said, holding out a hand to shake.*

*When Sophie took his hand, she felt a zing of electricity. She giggled—giggled! The Grown-Ass Woman giggled. It was too late, the giggle was out, and now he would think she was someone who giggled. She cleared her throat and took a deep breath to focus her mind, and said her name.*

*"I know." Bernard nodded, friendly and welcoming. Later, he would confess that he was dismissing her as out of his league, and that if he had actually thought he stood a chance with her, he'd have been a nervous wreck.*

*After the dinner, and throughout her time at the school, Sophie would pass Bernard in the hall with a friendly wave and smile, and there was always that same zing of electricity, the same butterflies.*

*"Why?" she asked the butterflies. "Why him?"*

*She had learned that Bernard was divorced, had kids, was therefore broke and laden with emotional baggage and had no time in his life for someone new. That was not what she was looking for. She was looking for laughter and travel and unencumbered fun.*

*The butterflies didn't care. "He has pretty eyes!" they enthused.*

*"There's a boy," she finally admitted to Emily. "And there are butterflies. And I don't understand because I*

*am a Grown-Ass Woman. I don't need this man and all his problems in my life."*

*Emily said, "Well, the science says—"*

*Sophie interrupted, "Emily Nagoski, you are not going to tell me the science says women need men. You, the feminist, the sex educator, the science nerd, are not going to tell me that science says women aren't complete without men."*

*"Oh geez, of course not!" Emily said.*

*"Good," Sophie said.*

*"But," Emily pressed, "the butterflies know something you don't."*

*This chapter is about what the butterflies know.*

"When you were little, who held you when you cried?"

That's the question therapist and researcher Sue Johnson asks her clients.

If she were a nutritionist, Sue might ask, "When you were little, what did you eat when you were hungry?"

People who grew up in a home where food was abundant, nourishing, and free of guilt and shame can answer that question with pleasure. People who grew up in homes where food was either scarce, low in quality, or laden with guilt and shame would answer it very differently, would feel very differently just thinking about it.

Social connection is a form of nourishment, like food. Just as our early experiences shape our present-day relationship with food, so our early experiences of connection shape our present-day relationships with other people. Our specific nutritional needs change over the course of our life-span, but the fundamental need for food does not; similarly, our need for connection changes across our life-spans, but our fundamental need for connection does not. And the culture we live in constrains the food choices available to us. Same goes for connection.

Being alone as an infant isn't just lonely; it's a matter of life and death—and it's not just that babies die if they aren't fed and kept warm and held out of reach of predatory carnivores. Babies can literally die of loneliness itself, even if their other needs are met.[1] Contact with another person is a basic biological need; loneliness is a form of starvation.

Even as adults, connection nourishes us in a literal, physiological way, regulating our heart rates and respiration rates, influencing the emotional activation in our brains, shifting our immune response to injuries and wounds, changing our exposure to stressors, and modulating our stress response.[2] We literally sicken and die without connection. A 2015 meta-analysis, encompassing seventy different studies and over three million research participants from around the globe, found that social isolation and loneliness increased a person's odds of an early death by 25 to 30 percent.[3] In describing the results of a 2018 study on the health impact of loneliness, a chief medical officer for an insurance company described loneliness as having "the same impact on mortality as smoking fifteen cigarettes a day."[4] Also in 2018, the United Kingdom's government created a Commission on Loneliness, framing it as a public health issue with the same health impact as living with a chronic disease like diabetes.[5] Residing in the beating heart of every adult human is that infant who will literally die if she isn't connected with other people.

And yet the "common wisdom" is that individual development should be a linear progression from dependence to autonomy. When psychologists began formulating theories about human development, they concluded that it's "immature" to depend on others. The best, strongest, sanest, smartest, and most grown-up people, they said, are the ones who don't need anyone to do anything for them.

Worse, Human Giver Syndrome says that path is not for everyone. Imagine an infant boy who learns to talk and walk and feed himself and control when he poops and pees; he learns to read and count and do chemistry; and he shifts from wanting to be held by his mommy to wanting to leave home and be independent, at which point he is a full-fledged human being. An infant girl, on the other hand, is supposed to grow independent up to a point, but then the next step is marriage and babies, at which point she is a full-fledged human giver. An identity grounded in autonomy is considered stronger, superior, and masculine. An identity grounded in connection is weaker, inferior, and feminine.

It remains popular wisdom that healthy people should feel 100 percent whole, with or without a romantic partner or the approval of others or the support of a family or community. Social connection should be a "bonus," not an essential component to our well-being—a supplement, not a staple. No wonder the first waves of feminists considered independence the ideal.

This is the heretical truth: No one is "complete" without other people—and we mean this literally. To be complete without social connection is to be nourished without food. It doesn't happen. We get hungry. We get lonely. We must feed ourselves or die. We don't mean you "need a man" or any kind of romantic partner. We mean you need connection in any or all of its varied forms. And it is also true that the lifelong development of autonomy is as innate to human nature as the drive to connect. We need *both* connection and autonomy. That's not a contradiction. Humans are built to *oscillate* from connection to autonomy and back again.

This chapter begins Part III: Wax On, Wax Off, where we describe daily choices and actions that will fight the causes of burnout—the enemies we named in Part II.

"Wax on, wax off," as Mr. Miyagi instructs Danny LaRusso in *The Karate Kid*. "Don't forget to breathe." Breathing: another cycle, another oscillation—breathe in . . . breathe out.

## "Connection" Is Literal

As twins, we have one pure talent, an ability bestowed on us from on high, with no training or effort on our part: the three-legged race. That's the children's field-day game where you tie one kid's left ankle to another kid's right ankle, and the pair runs down the field together, racing against other pairs of kids. At eight years old, we kicked ass at the three-legged race; we left everyone in the dust.

The same mechanism that allowed us to synchronize on the playground was also at work on the school bus: when one of us was being bullied and started to cry, the other started crying, too—seemingly out of the blue. We don't even remember which of us was being bullied. There was no string tying us to each other as there was on the playground; there was only the emotional attunement that synchronized our feelings. But that attunement and synchrony are as concrete, as real, as the string.

Science has just begun to be able to measure this phenomenon. Two-person neuroscience (2PN) is brand new and researchers are still trying to establish the most valid and effective ways to measure, in the brain, the experience of connected synchrony, but so far the results are astonishing.[6] When people watch a movie together, their brains' emotional responses synchronize, even if they're strangers. Simply sharing physical space with someone—mere co-presence—can be enough to synchronize heartbeats. We automatically mirror the facial expression of the person we're talking to and experience the emotion that goes with those expressions, and we involuntarily match body movements and vocal pitch.[7] We are all walking around co-regulating one another all the time, synchronizing without trying, without even necessarily being aware that it's happening.[8] Your internal state is profoundly contagious, and it is profoundly susceptible to "catching" the internal states of the people around you at work and at home and at the grocery store and on the bus.

This mutual co-regulation begins from the earliest moments

of our lives, and it shapes our brains.[9] The exchange of loving looks between infant and adult caregiver releases dopamine, a neuropeptide famous for bonding us with others and facilitating the growth of neural connections, while the exchange of negative looks between infant and caregiver releases cortisol, the infamous stress hormone, which disrupts the production of neural connections.[10] You spent the first two years of life assuming that what you felt was what everyone around you felt—checking in with the adults around you to see how they felt, and adopting their feelings as your own. Not by choice; by instinct. If the grown-up holding you is calm and relaxed, then your nervous system knows it can be calm and relaxed, too. If that grown-up is stressed and anxious, then there must be something to be anxious about, so your nervous system puts you in that state, too.[11]

By the age of two or three, a child still can't survive on her own, but she begins to understand that other people have internal experiences that are separate from hers. By adolescence, she might be able to survive on her own, but humans don't go off alone, the way many other animals do. We stay in social groups and develop mutual connections with our peers, which are shaped by the ways we connected (or, more technically, "attached") with our caregivers as infants.

Sharing space with anyone else means sharing energy—literally. Connection moves us at the level of our atoms. Each particle we are made of influences and is influenced by the particle next to it in an unending chain that exists on the smallest and largest scales you can imagine, and every scale in between. Swing a pendulum near another pendulum that's the same size, and they will gradually entrain, often swinging in the same direction at the same time. We're made of energy. The nature of energy is to be shared, to spread, to connect one thing to another. Sharing space with other people means that our energy influences theirs, and theirs influences ours. It's physics. And psychology. And unavoidable. And amazing.

And what does this do for us?

*It's easy to hear "Connection is important!" and think it means something intangible, like emotional connection, gal pals cheering you on, romantic partners listening and holding you while you cry, and hearing your kid say, "I love you." And it is that. Connection is a feeling.*

*But it's also pragmatic. Life is complicated and expensive and time-consuming. We need help.*

*Julie needed help. Her—oh, God—"bowel retraining" required, among other things, half an hour every day for—oh, God—"toilet time." To create that time, she had to offload some of the other things she was doing, things that still needed to get done, just not by her.*

*Her mom showed up for her; she cooked big meals on Sundays and brought them over, frozen, in containers. Diana's friends' parents showed up, helping with carpooling. To Julie's amazement, all her friends showed up. One friend spontaneously organized a shared calendar, where everyone volunteered to bring food on different days or take Diana out.*

*You know who else showed up? Her husband.*

*It's time to introduce you to Jeremy. Like Julie, he's an English teacher. He wrote his master's thesis on E. M. Forster. He has long eyelashes and intelligent brown eyes. When their daughter was obsessed with* Tangled, *he perfected a "smolder" look, just like Flynn Rider's, and it worked as well on Julie as on Diana. He always called the plumber or the contractor or whoever else needed to be called and scheduled and met to keep the house standing. And he loved Julie. He didn't understand how they had grown so far apart. All he knew is when he tried to help, he got scolded. So he stopped trying.*

*After Julie's poop episode, she sat down with him for a serious talk, despite her dread of the fight it could trigger.*

*She explained the situation (one of the benefits of a long-term intimate relationship is you get to a point where you can talk frankly about each other's poop), and she asked for what she needed: time.*

*He said, "Well, the house has to get cleaned. If we hired cleaners, we'd have to organize stuff before they come and I don't want the hassle. I can do it myself, if you'll just let me do it and not tell me how."*

*Connection isn't always warm and fuzzy. But Julie agreed.*

*He made Saturday cleaning day, and he turned it into a project he shared wth their daughter. The first Saturday afternoon Julie came home from a physical therapy appointment to find the house tidy—not tidy like she would have made it, but tidy, and she hadn't had to do it herself—she almost cried. There was food in the oven that she hadn't had to cook. All the people she cared about most were there for her. All she had to do to accept their help was let go of her impulse to be in control and make everything perfect.*

*Ha. "All."*

*Sometimes connection is emotional support. Sometimes it's information and education, like the medical professionals helping her relearn how to live in a body. And sometimes it's cooking, carpools, dishes, dusting, putting things back where they belong. Public health theory calls it "instrumental support."*

*To Julie, it just felt like "having a wife."*

## Good Connection Is Good for You

People vary in their appetites for connection.[12] Our variability is partly explained by introversion or extroversion, partly by the pleasure an individual experiences in socializing, and it also seems to be its own little quirk of personality.[13] Researchers can assess it as simply as asking a person whether they agree or disagree with the statement "I have a strong need to belong."[14] There is no "right amount" of needing to belong; there's just the amount of belonging that feels right for you.

Let's talk about the health benefits of getting the connection you need. Caveat: Connection is emphatically not just about marriagey-type relationships; it's about having positive relationships of all kinds, including friends, BFFLs, besties, buds, bros, and the fam. But spousal relationships might be the most commonly studied, so those are the ones that provide the most evidence of connection's benefits to our lives.

For example, a recent meta-analysis of more than seventy thousand participants (all in heterosexual marriages) across a dozen nations found that worse marital quality leads to worse physical health and shorter life, as well as declining mental health.[15] The standards for "quality" weren't intimidatingly high; they included "high self-reported satisfaction with the relationship, predominantly positive attitudes toward one's partner, and low levels of hostile and negative behavior." In short, "I'm satisfied with my relationship, I like my partner, and we're generally pretty supportive and nice to each other." But this baseline level of satisfaction can be powerful. Among people with higher marital quality, injuries and wounds heal faster and chronic pain interferes less with quality of life. In fact, relationship quality was found to be a better predictor of health than smoking, and smoking is among the strongest predictors of ill health. And the benefits of a high-quality relationship were sometimes even greater for women than for men.

Researchers found that this effect is probably due, at least in part, to the fact that people tend to take better care of themselves when they're in a high-quality relationship. In other words, our "self-care" is facilitated by the ways we care for and are cared for by someone else.

A loved one doesn't have to be your literal twin for it to happen to you. We hope you have at least one person in your life so attuned to you that they quite literally feel your pain, and stand with you inside it.

These energy-creating connections are what we call the "Bubble of Love."

## The Bubble of Love

Social connections fuel your body just as eating nutritious foods and taking deep breaths do.[16] If Human Giver Syndrome is a virus, the Bubble of Love is the environment that fuels your immune response. You might experience connection in the Bubble with one person at a time—that's Emily's most common experience. Or you might feel it most strongly in large, cooperative groups—which has been Amelia's experience. You might experience it best with your best friends. Your spouse. Your church family. Your dog—yes, we experience these kinds of connections with other species. Different Bubbles have different styles; you don't experience or express connection with your roller derby teammates the same way you would with your family, and you don't experience or express connection with your family the same way you would with your anti-capitalist, womynist knitting group—but all these different energy-creating Bubbles of Love share two specific ingredients: trust and connected knowing.

## Bubble Ingredient #1: Trust

Lots of species, including humans, keep track of who gives something to another and who reciprocates. The belief that the people around us will reciprocate in proportion to what we give them is called "trust."

Researchers, particularly in economic science but also in psychology, use the Trust Game as a tool for discovering the ways people respond to being trusted or not, being betrayed or not. If you want to know more about that science, just google "Trust Game." They use money. We're going to use cupcakes. The experiments go like this:

Researchers put Emily and Amelia in a lab. They give Amelia four cupcakes and a choice. She can take her cupcakes and go home, or she can give Emily any number of the cupcakes she chooses. Any cupcake she chooses to give Emily transforms into *three* cupcakes. So she can give away one cupcake, and Emily will get three while Amelia still has three. She can give away two, and Emily will have six while Amelia has two. And so on.

And then if Emily gets any cupcakes, she, too, has a choice. She can choose to return some to Amelia, or she can take her cupcakes and go home.

If Amelia trusts Emily, she gives away all four of her cupcakes, meaning a dozen cupcakes for Emily! If Emily is trustworthy, she gives half back, and they both get six! Trust followed by reciprocity results in maximum cupcakes and a peaceable queendom.

In real life, the "cupcakes" we give and receive in relationships can be almost anything—money, time, attention, actual cupcakes, or compassion for our difficult feelings. That last is the most important cupcake of all. If we turn toward someone with our difficult feelings—sadness, anger, hurt—and they tune in to our feelings without judgment or defensiveness, it helps us to move through that feeling, like a tunnel, to the light at the end.

This definition of trust can be boiled down to one question: "Are you there for me?"[17] Trustworthy people are there for each other, and that mutual trust and trustworthiness maximizes wellness for both people.

But suppose Emily is having PMS cravings at the moment, and twelve cupcakes look like dinner. She scarfs them down right there in the research lab, then runs out the door, leaving Amelia alone with zero cupcakes and a deep sense of betrayal.

This activates a stress response. Amelia may feel motivated, for example, to seek revenge. In reality, revenge is neither the usual nor the most productive response to betrayal. The most likely and valuable thing Amelia will do after Emily's betrayal is go home and complain to her husband that Emily took all the cupcakes! A supportive guy, he bakes her a batch of her own dozen cupcakes and invites some friends over, who all bring even more cupcakes and agree that Emily is a PMSing jerk. Emerging from the hormonal fog, eventually even Emily will agree, and she'll show up at Amelia's house with even more cupcakes, apologize, and agree not to do that again. In this way, trust is repaired and the Bubble is stabilized.[18]

However, if Emily says she's sorry but she just can't control her cupcake-swiping urges, Amelia may forgive her, but she would be wise to put Emily on the periphery of the Bubble.

Outside the energy-generating Bubble of Love, some jerk might say to Amelia, "That's what you get for giving away all your cupcakes." But that's why they're outside the Bubble. People who don't trust or are untrustworthy are energy drains.

Let's take a moment to explore the connection between trust and "authenticity."

Authenticity means "being totally yourself" and sharing the most intimate parts of yourself, including the parts people might judge.[19] Being authentic requires trust, knowing that the person with whom you share these potentially rejectable thoughts and feelings will not betray you. A lot of self-help books (and, notably, a lot of books on marketing and sales) promote authenticity.

But strategic *inauthenticity* is part of trust, too.[20] Sometimes you go to your kid's best friend's birthday party even though your ex will also be there, and you smile and make socially acceptable conversation, because that's what you want your kid to remember about the day. You don't want her to remember that time you threw her best friend's birthday cake in your ex's face while screaming like a banshee.

Polite, socially acceptable suppression of our rage is "inauthentic," insofar as we are not sharing our full selves. And that is part of trust, too. Part of being trustworthy is meeting expectations and staying in line, as if you were a well-behaved woman.

Authenticity comes on the phone that evening, when you tell your best friend how well you behaved, despite the desire to kick the table over and go full Hulk. It comes when you cry as you say your kid will probably never know how hard you had to work, that the whole point of all that hard work was so that she would never need to know how hard you had to work.

And your best friend receives the cupcakes of your difficult emotions and returns them to you by saying, "But *I* know how hard you worked, and I am proud of you. And what is your plan to purge all that rage your body is still holding?"

When the people in our Bubble can turn with kindness and compassion toward our difficult emotions, and we can do the same for them, it strengthens the Bubble like nothing else.

## Bubble Ingredient #2: Connected Knowing

Blythe McVicker Clinchy codified two divergent ways of knowing: "separate knowing" and "connected knowing."

In separate knowing, you separate an idea from its context and assess it in terms of some externally imposed rules—rules that have proven to be immensely powerful as a tool for scientific advancement. Still, it's easy to read her 1996 description of a "separate knower" and think, with our twenty-first-century social-media brains: "mansplainer":

> *If you approach this chapter as a separate knower, you examine its arguments with a critical eye, insisting that I justify every point . . . looking for flaws in my reasoning, considering how I might be misinterpreting the evidence I present, what alternative interpretations could*

*be made, and whether I might be omitting evidence that would contradict my position.*[21]

And immediately, she points out the crucial strength of separate knowing:

*The standards you apply in evaluating my arguments are objective and impersonal; they have been agreed upon and codified by logicians and scientists.*

There's a reason your entire formal education was likely devoted to training you in separate knowing. Separate knowing winnows the wheat from the chaff.

*Connected knowing,* in contrast, involves coming to understand an idea by exploring it within its context. You put yourself in the shoes of the other person, to try on their point of view. You suspend (temporarily) your doubts, judgments, criticisms, and personal needs, in favor of exploring their perspective—not because you accept it, but because you want to understand. Then you bring in elements of your own life experience or personality, holding these up to the other point of view, testing it and turning it and testing it again, exploring what it would be like to have this person's perspective, within your own point of view. Sometimes we experience the process of connected knowing as a morphing or reshaping of ourselves into the form that fits the other person—like trying on someone else's clothes. In the process, you feel how comfortable (or uncomfortable) it would be for you to have the same perspective.

It's called "connected knowing" because it doesn't separate an idea from its context; it insists that we can only understand something if we also understand how it relates to the context it comes from. If separate knowing separates wheat from chaff, connected knowing explores the relationship between the wheat and the chaff, seeking to understand where each comes from and why they accompany each other.

Though everyone uses both, women are more likely to use connected knowing than separate knowing, and the opposite is true for men.[22]

Perhaps because of this difference, connected knowing is often dismissed as "irrational," as if the only alternative to the scientific method and logical reasoning is nonsense. It's not. Connected knowing is careful, effortful, often slow, and *intensely rational*, meaning it follows predictable patterns and progression. It integrates emotion into the information needed to understand an idea. It's also imaginative, requiring the listener to *suspend* their emotional reactions to differences and allow themselves to try on a viewpoint distinct from their own.

But the most energy-cresting characteristic of connected knowing is that it isn't just a way to connect with and understand others; it's a way to connect with and understand our own internal experience and develop our own identities, through connection with others.

Women, more so than men, build our identities within the context of our relationships. We don't know why this difference exists—Are we born that way? Do we learn it from our culture? Who knows?—but for our purposes, it doesn't matter why. What matters is that connected knowing fosters both healthy relationships and healthy individual identity. Connected knowing is why women often find profound satisfaction in understanding themselves and their identity in terms of their relationships—sister, daughter, mother, friend.

Of course, insisting that women can *only* develop their identities within relationships is just another way of imposing gendered rules that limit women's access to other sources of growth, as well as to basic autonomy. But if we insist women "should" develop their identities within the pursuit of "achievement" rather than through relationships, we're pathologizing women's (and every human's) innate search for themselves through connection. Knowing yourself better by learning about others is healthy. Neither is right or wrong, good or bad, and people vary in the degree to which they practice both ways of knowing. Again (and again), we need both; we need the freedom to move into and out of connection.

The blend of connected and separate knowing is "constructed knowing." This book is, by necessity, a product of constructed knowing, integrating separate and connected knowing into a textured whole. Emily and Amelia can try to learn and explain everything science has to say about the brain's and body's responses to stress—separate knowing—but we can never know what it feels like to be *you*, nor can we predict what's going to be effective in your life for dealing with the stress. Only *you* are the expert in you, so we've included stories and experiences from as many sources as possible, hoping you'll try them on as you read, see how they fit, and consider how you may accept or reject any given idea—connected knowing. Between the three of us— Emily, Amelia, and you, reader—we'll find our way to a plan that will work for you, even if it wouldn't work for anyone else.

## Signs You Need to Recharge in the Bubble of Love

In chapter 1, we described four signs that you need to stop dealing with your stressors and just deal with the stress itself. Here we'll describe four signs that you have to disengage from your autonomous efforts and seek connection. Each of these emotions is a different form of hunger for connection—that is, they're all different ways of feeling lonely:

*When you have been gaslit.* When you're asking yourself, "Am I crazy, or is there something completely unacceptable happening right now?" turn to someone who can relate; let them give you the reality check that yes, the gaslights are flickering.

*When you feel "not enough."* No individual can meet all the needs of the world. Humans are not built to do big things alone. We are built to do them *together.* When you experience the empty-handed feeling that you are just one person, unable to meet all the demands the world makes on you, helpless in the face of the endless, yawning need you see around you, recognize that emotion for what it is: a form of loneliness. Find your people. Call your friends and commiserate; consume all the YOU GO, GIRL! social media memes you like; watch *Wonder Woman* or *Hidden Figures* or *Moana* or whatever immerses you in a story of women working with a team of men, a team of women, or nature and the divine itself.

*When you're sad.* In the animated film *Inside Out*, the emotions in the head of a tween girl, Riley, struggle to cope with the exigencies of growing up. Joy, the emotions' leader, tries to contain Sadness, to keep her from getting in the way. Joy literally draws a circle on the floor and tells Sadness to stay inside the circle. That's the way many of us have been taught to treat our sadness: keep it under control, because it makes others uncomfortable. (Because, again: human givers.)

But at the critical turning point, when Joy is in a pit of despair, on the verge of giving up all hope, she remembers the day Riley missed the winning shot of her hockey game. On the verge of quitting, Riley sat alone, until her parents came to talk to her. They led her to her team, who embraced her.

"Sadness," Joy whispers in revelation. "Mom and Dad . . . the team . . . They came to help *because of Sadness.*"

Sadness is the beacon; it is the Bat-Signal. Though many of us were taught that we should mask our uncomfortable emotions, the truth about sadness is that we find our way out of that tunnel most efficiently when we have a friend who calls through the darkness, "I'm right here!" or better yet, someone who can take our hand in the dark and say, "Any step we take *together* is a step toward the light."

*When you are boiling with rage.* Rage has a special place in women's lives and a special role in the Bubble of Love. More, even, than sadness, many of us have been taught to swallow our rage, hide it even from ourselves. We have been taught to fear rage—our own, as well as others'—because its power can be used as a weapon. *Can* be. A chef's knife can be used as a weapon. And it can help you prepare a feast. It's all in how you use it. We don't want to hurt anyone, and rage is indeed very, very powerful.

Bring your rage into the Bubble with your loved ones' permission, and complete the stress response cycle with them. If your Bubble is a rugby team, you can leverage your rage in a match or practice. If your Bubble is a knitting circle, you might need to get creative. Use your body. Jump up and down, get noisy, release all that energy, share it with others.

"Yes!" say the people in your Bubble. "That was some bullshit you dealt with!"

Rage gives you strength and energy and the urge to fight, and sharing that energy in the Bubble changes it from something potentially dangerous to something safe and potentially transformative.

---

### ÜBER-BUBBLE

For eight years, Emily worked as the health educator at Smith College, a campus crowded with Lisa Simpsons: highly intelligent, high-achieving women, who are also intensely driven, ambitious, hardworking, sensitive, and social justice–minded. Many struggle with anxiety, depression, disordered eating, or self-harm. And Emily was their health educator.

In 2014, she gave a talk titled "Love Is an Open Door: *Frozen* and the Science of 'the Feels,'" in which she explained the science of emotion, as illustrated by that year's Disney blockbuster, *Frozen*.

Emily asked Amelia's musical advice. "Should I play recordings from the movie? Would it be better to ask a music professor if she has students who could perform the songs live?"

"Make it a sing-along," Amelia said. "Let them do the singing."

She did, and it turned out to be the highlight of Emily's time at Smith.

Three hundred students attended on a Friday evening in September. Half an hour in, right at the midpoint of the talk, Emily played the video of "Let It Go," complete with lyrics at the bottom of the screen.

Hundreds of driven, brilliant, perfectionistic women belted out, "That perfect girl is gone!" The sound filled the entire Campus Center. You could hear it on the lawn outside. It was breathtaking. Emily looked at the sea of upturned faces, lit by the larger-than-life video of Queen Elsa fully expressing her power for the first time in her life, and thought, *How do we get them to do this every day?* After that talk, students approached Emily in tears, telling her that was exactly what they needed—and nobody was saying the science part of the talk was what they needed. It was the singing.

This is what we call Über-Bubble, and you make it with rhythmic play, including music-making. It happens to singers in a choir, players on a team, voters on election night amid a group of likeminded supporters, or even moviegoers in a crowd of strangers who share enthusiasm for *Black Panther*. In these activities, through synchronous rhythmic movement, through song, through play, through intense effort to achieve a shared goal, for a few moments we step onto a neurological bridge, and the barrier between us and other people dissolves—sometimes a lot, sometimes just a little—and we experience our own identity as something that extends beyond our skin, into the intangible "Us." Über-Bubble.

Über-Bubble doesn't just feel good; it actively increases cooperation within a group.[23] Laurel Trainor at the McMaster Institute of Music and the Mind has demonstrated that toddlers who experience synchronous bouncing with another person are much more likely to help that person when she drops a pencil a few minutes later than babies who are bounced asynchronously with that person.[24] Adults who tap their fingers in time with a stranger are three times more likely to volunteer to help that person with a math and logic questionnaire than if they tap asynchronously.[25]

The pleasure of synchronized movement is built into our biology, and it's a powerful tool to access your greatest well-being.

*When we share trust, authenticity, and connected knowing with someone, we change, and it's scary and good and important. We come to know certain people, the right people, as intimately as we know ourselves, and, in coming to know them, we come to know ourselves in new and deeper ways. Sophie's butterflies knew that Bernard was one of those people.*

*But because Bernard was not what she was looking for, Sophie declined his invitations to dinner and movies and various other date-like activities. She became friends with him, though, almost against her will. He was funny and smart and warmhearted and a great dad, and he listened to her in a way that made her know herself better.*

*"It's extremely inconvenient!" Sophie said to Emily.*

*"Positive reappraisal!" Emily answered. "When it's inconvenient, it's probably doing the most for you."*

*We don't need other people's love in order to love ourselves; we don't need a romantic partner to be "complete." But we need other people to teach us how to love ourselves best.*

*At last, Sophie let herself dive in, and her world transformed. She said, "I thought love would just be like being me, plus knowing that if I'm bleeding to death somebody will call an ambulance. But it's more than that. I see myself in his eyes, and I find new ways to know and love myself, at the same time that I find new ways to know and love him, and then I know and love us and what we are together, which is this thing beyond what either of us is."*

*Then she started using phrases like "emergent properties of complex dynamical systems," and Emily nodded in excitement, and from there it got technical.*

*The point is connection is good for us. It is not weakness; it doesn't mean we're "needy." It makes us stronger.*

We saw in chapter 1 that positive social interaction and affection complete the cycle. Here in chapter 6, we're declaring connection to be as primary a source of strength as any basic biological need.

In the next chapter, we'll talk about an equally important source of strength: rest.

## tl;dr:

- Connection—with friends, family, pets, the divine, etc.—is as necessary as food and water. Humans are not built to function autonomously; we are built to oscillate between connection and autonomy and back again.

- We are all constantly "co-regulating" one another without even being aware it's happening—synchronizing heartbeats, changing moods, and helping one another feel seen and heard.

- Certain kinds of connection create energy. When you share mutual trust and "connected knowing" with someone, you co-create energy that renews both people. We call this the "Bubble of Love."

- Sadness, rage, and the feeling that you are not "enough" are forms of loneliness. When you experience these emotions, connect.

# 7

# WHAT MAKES YOU STRONGER

*Julie was still tired, but bowel retraining meant that she finally accepted help. Lots of it. Help she had needed for years but had been too, maybe, proud, to ask for? Whatever the reason, she had held on to the idea that she was supposed to do all of it herself . . . right up until the moment when "all of it" broke her body.*

*So now she was making like Queen Elsa and letting it go.*

*Vindication, of a kind, and deeper insight, came when Jeremy volunteered to take on Diana Duty when his school was on spring break but neither Diana's nor Julie's schools were.*

*He learned a lot about his daughter that week. He discovered that she had unshakable opinions about what*

*she should wear, and they were not always ideas that con-
formed to Jeremy's standards or, indeed, to the school
dress code. Jeremy had not known about the dress code
until the school called to tell him to bring clothes for his
daughter to change into. Diana also had opinions about
what she ate, and they were not opinions that conformed
to any nutritional guidelines of which Jeremy was aware.
Vegetables? No. Fruit? Only in the form of a roll-up or
gummy, please. He cooked, and she wouldn't eat, and
they argued, and he felt like an asshole, his stomach
churning from anger and frustration and worry.*

*And the time it took! The shuttling to and from les-
sons, the negotiations, the monitoring to make sure everything got done that needed to get done, the repetition, the
repetition, God help him, the repetition.*

*But more than the time, the emotional drain! The en-
forced patience, the reasoning and instruction, the constant management of his own frustration, trying to be
the loving, happy, patient father he wanted to be, while
counting the hours until spring break was over.*

*At the end of the week, he sat at the kitchen table, one
palm on his forehead, as he described the week. He looked
up at Julie for some sympathy and found her smiling at
him, relaxed and amused. It distracted him from his tirade.*

*"You look better. I mean, you look good."*

*Julie raised her eyebrow at him.*

*"I just mean you look not bothered."*

*Julie acknowledged his point. "That's true. A lot of
times, I haven't been able to handle your stuff when I was
all stressed out, and then you were unloading your stress
on me, too." She sent her attention to her body, tuning in
to what it was experiencing at that moment, and said,
"At this moment, I feel like I can handle it."*

*This chapter is about where Julie got that strength.*

Nietzsche (ugh) told us, "What doesn't kill you makes you stronger."

You've been hearing this for years, in one form or another, but let's be specific. Like, if you're hit by a car and don't die, does *the car* make you stronger? No. Does injury or disease make you stronger? No. Does suffering alone build character? No. These things leave you more vulnerable to further injury.

What makes you stronger is whatever happens to you *after* you survive the thing that didn't kill you.

What makes you stronger is *rest*.

Rest is, quite simply, when you stop using a part of you that's used up, worn out, damaged, or inflamed, so that it has a chance to renew itself. And it's the topic of this chapter.

"Rest" doesn't just mean sleep—though of course sleep is essential. Rest also includes switching from one type of activity to another. Mental energy, like stress, has a cycle it runs through, an oscillation from task focus to processing and back to task focus. The idea that you can use "grit" or "self-control" to stay focused and productive every minute of every day is not merely incorrect, it is gaslighting, and it is potentially damaging your brain.

Let's take a moment to wrap our brains around this strange reality: Life in the modern developed world is such that many of us have a vast overabundance of virtually everything . . . yet often we can't meet our basic, life-sustaining, physiological needs without feeling guilty, ashamed, lazy, greedy, conflicted, or, at best, defiant. An Internet meme we like goes, "You don't have to set yourself on fire to keep other people warm." But according to Human Giver Syndrome, you definitely *should*. As "human givers," women live with the expectation that we *give* every part of our humanity, including our bodies, our health, and our very lives. Our time, energy, and attention should go toward someone *else's* well-being, not be squandered on our own. What's the matter with you, you lazy, selfish monster, sleeping seven hours a night? *Get back in line,* with the rest of us exhausted, righteous givers.

Toward the end of this chapter, you'll read our science-based conclusion about just how much rest it takes for you to survive and grow stronger, and you may scoff and say, "I don't have time for that!" or "That's too extreme!" and maybe that's true. . . . But maybe that's just what Human Giver Syndrome wants you to believe. Maybe, to get enough rest to keep yourself fully functional, you're going to have to choose your own well-being— your own *life*—over the demands of Human Giver Syndrome.

As Audre Lorde put it, "Caring for myself is not self-indulgence, it is self-preservation, and that is an act of political warfare." This chapter is about arming you for that battle— a battle that is quite literally a fight for your life. We offer the best available scientific evidence to help you build a practice of sustainable living, to protect you from the toxic cultural narrative of self-destruction as virtue.

So curl up someplace cozy, and let's talk about rest.

## Default Mode—aka Daydreaming

We are built to oscillate between work and rest. When we allow for this oscillation, the quality of our work improves, along with our health.

To illustrate: In one study, a group of research participants were asked to write down whatever thoughts they had, but were explicitly told they should try not to write about a white bear. This was effortful enough to deplete some mental energy. Then half the participants were instructed to relax as much as they could between tasks—the researchers even played a Satie piano piece to reinforce the idea that they should be relaxing—while the other half were given no instructions and just sat there waiting for the next task. Result? The group that relaxed persisted twice as long at the next depleting task (a set of three-digit multiplication problems) than the group that simply waited.[1] Conclusion: Rest makes us more persistent and productive.

How?

A growing body of research has established that we do our best at any given task for only a limited amount of time, energy, or attention, then our performance drops off, our attention wanders, and our motivation evaporates.[2]

But *resting* after a depleting activity eliminates the effects of fatigue.[3]

When you drop out of task-focused attention and into neutral, your "resting" brain is not doing nothing—far from it. In fact, there's very little difference in the amount of energy used by your brain when you're in the middle of doing your taxes and when you're standing at the counter, mind wandering while you wait to be handed your takeout order.[4]

Running in the background of your awareness is what neuroscientists call the "default mode network," a collection of linked brain areas that function as a kind of low-grade dreaming when your attention is not focused on a task.[5] When your mind is "wandering," your default mode network is online. It assesses your present state and it plans for the future, a little like a chess-playing computer, rapidly scanning the board and running simulations to see what would happen if you made a particular move. And it's doing it without active intervention from you.

Life coach extraordinaire Martha Beck figured this out without the science. When her team is struggling at the office, the solution is to stop working, turn off their computers, and go play or rest. Where so many others would "dig in," set up a command central and not stop until a solution was found, she asks her team to take a break.

"It works every time," Beck told *Bloomberg Businessweek*.[6] "I don't know why, but it does, so I guess I don't really need to know."

The default mode network is why. (Also, some team members

are probably completing their stress response cycles during the breaks, which allows them to be more creative and curious.)

Research on this network is very new and lots of questions remain unanswered about exactly what it does and how it works, but it's increasingly clear that the more balanced the linkages between the different domains of the default mode network are, and the more fluidly a person can toggle from default to attentive, the more creative, socially skilled, and happy a person is likely to be.[7]

Mental rest is not idleness; it is the time necessary for your brain to process the world.[8] So, for example, while writing this book, Emily would write for an hour or two, then go put in a load of laundry or dishes. Write for another hour or two and then empty the dishwasher or rotate the laundry. In the same way the laundry was running while Emily wrote, her default mode was running while she folded towels. The default mode network didn't need her help—in fact, it needed her to stop writing, so that it could work on the puzzle she had given it, without her looking over its shoulder. Then when she came back to work, her default mode would hand her new insight. If she had stayed chained to her desk, insisting that she couldn't move until she had reached a certain word count, she may have written more words, but they would have been lower-quality words.

And sometimes Emily wasn't folding laundry like a good little housewife, she was playing a game on her phone, and that was fine, too, because what her brain needed was any low-demand task that allowed her default mode to come online.

Walking away from a task or a problem doesn't mean you're "quitting" or giving up. It means you're recruiting *all* your brain's processes for a particular task—including the capabilities that don't involve your effortful attention.

Not everyone slips comfortably into default mode. This has been tested empirically in a series of fairly hilarious studies:[9]

Researchers first asked participants to experience a mild electrical shock, along with various other pleasant or unpleasant stimuli.

"Would you pay five dollars never to have to feel that shock again?" the researchers asked.

"Hellz yes," the participant would say.

Then they took the participant into a quiet room that contained the electric shock device, and left them alone, with instructions to "entertain themselves with their thoughts" for fifteen minutes.

"The shock machine is here. You can touch it or not, it's up to you," they told the participant who had just said they'd pay money not to feel that shock again.

In fact, a quarter of the women and two-thirds of the men gave themselves an electric shock rather than simply sit there and "just think." On average, they self-administered one or two shocks over the fifteen minutes.

Instead of being in default mode, research suggests these self-zapping participants were *bored*. Boredom is the discomfort you experience when your brain is in active-attention mode, but can't latch on to anything to attend to.[10] They were zapping themselves in desperation for something, anything, to pay attention to, even if it was uncomfortable.

Fortunately, there is *active rest*.

## Active Rest

Everybody knows a muscle that isn't used will atrophy. We all know a muscle that is worked constantly, without rest, will grow fatigued and eventually fail in exhaustion. And we all know a muscle that gets worked and rested and worked and rested will grow stronger.

But suppose you break your right leg, and while it's healing in a cast, you exercise your left leg. The signal from the left leg travels up the spine and crosses from one side to the other, sparking growth in the right leg—not as much as in the left, but enough to prevent some of the atrophy of disuse.[11] This is the original meaning of "cross-training"—literally, training across the spine.

But look, it's even bigger than that: When you work your muscles—especially your biggest muscles—you strengthen not just the muscles you're using but also your lungs and liver and brain. Exercising one part of you strengthens all of you; exercising the strongest parts of you strengthens the rest of you most efficiently. The same goes for cognitive, emotional, and social effort.

This is active rest: working one gear while resting the others.

So for example, sometimes the "rest" Emily's brain needed was not a low-demand task like laundry or YouTube, but a different kind of writing. Result: She wrote a novel at the same time as writing this book. Amelia worked full-time as a professor of music *and* conducted a children's choir, while writing the book. Most women are at least this productive—they rest certain gears while they work others, and this "active rest" makes us better at all the things we do.

People vary, including in what rest looks like for them.

But one universal need is sleep.

## Why Sleep?

Sleep is really strange. How can it make sense that we lay our bodies down and lose awareness of the outside world for hours at a time, while who knows what lions and hippos and other threats may be lurking? During certain phases of sleep, our motor functioning is locked off, so that our bodies can't respond to our brain's activation. There we lie, in the dark, paralyzed, unresponsive, and limp to the bone, as our eyeballs ticktock behind our closed lids and our attention is funneled away from the outside world toward an intense, multisensory hallucination—

a dream—that feels both real and urgent in the moment but will be forgotten by the waking mind within seconds of rousing.

Humans are designed to spend a third of their lives in this most vulnerable state—eight hours a day, every single day.

How can it make sense?

It turns out that the physiological, cognitive, emotional, and social benefits of spending a third of our lives unconscious outweigh even the costs in time, opportunity to do other things, and inattention to threats. Our whole body, including our brain, is working hard as we sleep, to accomplish life-preserving tasks that can be best achieved when we're not around to interfere. Quite simply, we are not complete without sleep.

Physical activity is not complete without sleep. While you sleep, your bones, blood vessels, digestive system, muscles (including your heart), and all your other body tissues heal from the damage you inflicted on them during the day. If you engaged in physical activity, your body will repair itself and grow stronger while you sleep. Physical activity without sleep, by contrast, leaves you more vulnerable to injury and illness than you would have been without the activity. If you're not going to sleep, better not exercise.

Learning is not complete without sleep. Your memories consolidate and new information is integrated into existing knowledge. Studying for a test, memorizing a speech, or learning a language? Review right before bed, then sleep for seven to nine hours. Your brain will soak up the information like grass absorbing rain after a drought. Any motor skills you practiced—skiing or playing piano or walking up the stairs—get integrated, so that you're better at them the next day. The benefits of practice come not during the practice itself but during sleep; without it, your skill will actually decline, no matter how much you practice. If you're not going to sleep, you're studying and practicing for nothing.

Emotions are not complete without sleep. You can dream about beating the daylights out of your enemy, and you'll wake up feeling released from the grip of your rage, better able to handle interpersonal conflict. In one study, professionals who got inadequate sleep were rated by their peers and their employees as having lower emotional intelligence.[12] Marital satisfaction, too, is linked to sleep quality.[13] Recent lack of sleep not only worsens conflict between spouses, it also heightens each person's inflammatory immune response to conflict, a biological marker paralleling each partner's heightened reactivity to their spouse's complaint.[14] If you're not getting adequate sleep, better avoid talking to other humans.

Did we say this yet? Sleep is *important*.

We are built to oscillate between wakefulness and sleep, because we require the things our brain does on its own during sleep to make us fully functional while we're awake.

And at its most extreme, sleep deprivation is a form of torture.[15] You can quite literally die of sleep deprivation—by physiological deprivation akin to starvation.[16] When researchers deprive rats of sleep for two weeks, the rats' immune systems become so impaired their blood becomes infected with their own gut bacteria and they die of septicemia.

"When you are broken, go to bed," goes the French proverb. You are not complete without sleep.

And what are the costs of inadequate sleep?

Inadequate sleep damages your physical health: chronic sleep deprivation—short sleep and disturbed sleep—is a causal factor in 20 percent of serious car accidents,[17] and in every common cause of death, including heart disease, cancer, diabetes, hypertension, Alzheimer's, and immune dysfunction, increasing risk by up to 45 percent.[18] Poor sleep is a better predictor of developing type 2 diabetes than lack of physical activity, but when was the last time anyone told you to get enough sleep to prevent diabetes?[19]

Inadequate sleep impairs brain functioning, including working memory and long-term memory, attention, decision-making, hand-eye coordination, calculation accuracy, logical reasoning, and creativity.[20] People who've been awake for nineteen hours (say, woke up at 7 A.M. and now it's 2 A.M.) are as impaired in their cognitive and motor functioning as a person who is legally intoxicated.[21] People who've slept just four hours the previous night are similarly impaired, as are those who've slept six or fewer hours every night for the last two weeks. Anything you wouldn't do drunk—drive, lead a work meeting, raise a child—don't try it if you've been awake for nineteen hours, slept only four hours the previous night, or slept fewer than six hours every night for two weeks.

Your social life is also affected by lack of sleep: team communication in the workplace and group decision-making are impaired, while hostility and even unethical workplace behavior increase.[22] Your emotional life is impacted, too: depression and sleep difficulties are closely intertwined, each exacerbating the other,[23] and insomnia predicts suicidal thoughts, even in people without depression.[24] Anxiety and sleep, too, are closely related and mutually causal.[25] If you struggle with depression, anxiety, or other mental health issues—which more than twice as many women as men do (a conservative estimate is about one in five women in their lifetime[26])—*sleep is medicine* for you.

This is not an area of research where there's any reasonable debate; the medical opinion is in: Sleep is good for you, and not sleeping is bad for you in every way—dangerous and potentially lethal. Three recent meta-analyses, comprising millions of research participants, found overall around a 12 percent greater risk of all-cause mortality among those who slept fewer than five or six hours a night.[27] If you make only one change in your life after reading this book, let it be getting more sleep.

## CAN YOU GET "TOO MUCH" SLEEP?

"But naps make me feel worse!" you may say.

When we're sleep deprived, our bodies try to compensate by activating the stress response—doses of adrenaline and cortisol to help us survive the temporary stressor of too little sleep—which masks the fatigue and impairment. The result is that sleep deprivation can act a little like alcohol; just as a person who has been drinking may be too impaired to know how impaired they are ("I'm fine, gimme the keys!"), a person who isn't rested may be too sleep deprived to be aware of how sleep deprived they are.

The counterintuitive result is that when we eventually sleep, the stress response reduces, so when we're actually better rested, we may *feel* less rested. Adrenaline is no longer masking our fatigue. And we groan, "Ugh, I slept too much," the way we'd groan after a huge meal, "Ugh, I ate too much."

Can you actually sleep "too much"?

The general rule is: If you're sleeping more than nine hours out of every twenty-four, and you still don't feel rested, that could be a sign of an underlying issue, and it would be good to talk with a medical provider.[28]

One day Emily said this to a group of students and one raised her hand and said, "But I've been sleeping, like, ten hours a night and I'm exhausted." Lots of people in the group had an opinion about what might be causing her exhaustion—everything from depression to narcolepsy to laziness—but Emily said, "If you're sleeping more than nine hours every night and don't feel rested, what do you do?"

"Talk to a doctor?" the student parroted back.

"Right."

Six months later, that student approached Emily and said, "Hey, you probably don't remember, but I'm the one who was sleeping ten—"

"Oh, I remember," Emily said.

"Well, I actually did go to the doctor and I did a sleep study, and it turned out I had really severe sleep apnea. Over the summer I had my tonsils and adenoids removed and now I sleep with a mask, and it has completely changed my life. I had no idea how sleep-deprived I was my whole life."

Bottom line: If you're sleeping more than nine hours a day and don't feel rested, talk to a medical provider.[29] And if you're thinking, "But Emily and Amelia, I'm trying. I give myself an eight-hour window of opportunity to sleep and the sleep doesn't happen! I literally can't get the sleep I need," talk to a medical provider. Do a sleep study. It could change your life. Maybe even save it.

## An "Invisible Workplace"

Sleep is a miracle. What else but sleep can mend a broken bone and a broken heart? What else but sleep leads us to a lost memory and to a new idea? What else but sleep can transform the damage done to our bodies, whether by a nice, long run or by trauma, into even greater strength?

Yet moral judgment about sleep is built into the cultural history of the West. Medieval theologians believed humans' need for sleep was "a divine punishment for the fall of man and a daily reminder to mankind of their sinfulness, weakness and imperfection."[30] America's puritanical forebears warned (incorrectly) that "immoderate sleep" could cause everything from seizures to infertility to poverty.[31] By the 1830s, medical journals were saying that more than four hours of sleep was "an intemperance."[32] Sloth.

The immorality of adequate sleep has changed somewhat over

the last fifty years. These days, the message is not so much that we don't need sleep, but that if a person has time to sleep, they're doing something wrong; they're not working hard enough. We've made a virtue of being exhausted, of denying ourselves rest. This idea is so embedded in the culture that Emily has lost count of the number of women who tell her they feel guilty about sleeping.

*Guilty*. About *sleeping*.

"How come?" Emily asked one group. "You may as well feel guilty about breathing! It's *necessary*. So why the guilt over sleep?"

"It's selfish," a woman answered. "When you're asleep, you're only helping yourself."

That woman was eighteen years old, and already a committed human giver.

As we've seen, sleep is essential not only for your own personal health, but also for your emotional health and relationships, so it's not even remotely "selfish." But the lesson here is: Human Giver Syndrome messes with women's sleep.

So no wonder sleep problems are more common in women than men, especially around menopause.[33] As researchers write, women's sleep is "an 'invisible workplace' in which they remain on duty throughout the night, available to provide the physical and emotional support needed to ensure the well-being of their family." And it's not limited to the inevitable insomnia-fest that is caring for a newborn, during which, of course, mothers in heterosexual couples are much more likely than fathers to interrupt their sleep to care for a child; this persists through the preschool years, regardless of which partner has a full-time job.[34] As human givers, women are expected to sacrifice their sleep for the benefit of others. So we deprive ourselves of a basic physiological need—not a lot, necessarily, but every day, over and over—and the accumulating deprivation wears us down, day by day, until there's too little left to do all the other things life expects of us.

It's not just cultural messages that make accessing sleep and rest difficult. Suppose you deal with all your stressors, you check all the boxes on your to-do list, and give yourself permission and opportunity to rest. If you've dealt with the stressors but haven't dealt with the stress itself, your brain won't let you rest. It will constantly scan for the lion that's about to come after you, so when you try to go to sleep, your brain won't let you fall asleep, or it will wake you up over and over, checking for that lion. Complete the cycle, so your brain can transition into rest.

## Forty-Two Percent

So how much rest is "adequate"?

Science says: 42 percent.

That's the percentage of time your body and brain need you to spend resting. It's about ten hours out of every twenty-four. It doesn't have to be every day; it can average out over a week or a month or more. But yeah. That much.

"That's ridiculous! I don't have that kind of time!" you might protest—and we remind you that we predicted you might feel that way, back at the start of the chapter.

We're not saying you *should* take 42 percent of your time to rest; we're saying if you don't take the 42 percent, the 42 percent will take you. It will grab you by the face, shove you to the ground, put its foot on your chest, and declare itself the victor.

Have you ever come down with a terrible cold as soon as you finished a huge project? Have you found yourself sleeping twelve or fourteen hours every day for the first three days of vacation? Have you, like Amelia, literally ended up in the hospital after a prolonged period of extreme stress? We've established by now that stress is a physiological phenomenon that impacts every system and function in our bodies, including immune functioning, digestive functioning, and hormones. To keep all of those systems in full working order, our biology requires that we spend 42 percent of our lives maintaining the organism of our physical existence.

Here's what your 42 percent might look like:

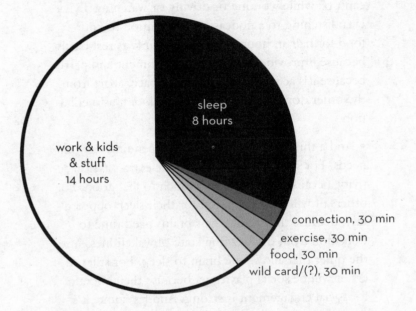

• Eight hours of sleep opportunity, give or take an hour.

• Twenty to thirty minutes of "stress-reducing conversation" with your partner or other trusted loved one.

• Thirty minutes of physical activity. Whether with people or alone, you do it with the explicit mindset of gear-switching, Feels-purging, rest-getting freedom. Physical activity counts as "rest" partly because it improves the quality of your sleep and partly because it completes the stress response cycle, transitioning your body out of a stressed state and into a resting state.

• Thirty minutes of paying attention to food. "Thirty minutes?" you say. Don't fret. That includes all meals, shopping, cooking, and eating, and it doesn't have to be all at once. It can be with people or alone, but it can't be while working or driving or watching TV or even listening to a podcast. Pay attention to your food for half an hour a day. This counts as rest partly because it provides necessary nourishment and partly because it's active rest, a change of pace, apart from the other domains of your life. Think of it as meditation.

• And a thirty-minute wild card, depending on your needs. For some people, this will be extra physical activity, because they need that much to feel good. For others, it will be preparation for their sleep opportunity, because they know their brains need time to transition from the buzzing state of wakefulness into the quiet that allows the brain to sleep. For still others, it will be social play time, because their appetite for social engagement is strong. And for some, it's simply a buffer for travel and changing clothes and other rest-preparation time (because: reality) during which you engage your default mode network—that is, you let your mind wander.

These are just averages, and as you can see, you'll sometimes do more than one thing at a time. Some people need more sleep than others—sleep need is estimated to be about 40 percent genetically heritable, so even identical twins can vary a lot.[35] Emily needs seven and a half hours, but Amelia needs nine, and if she only gets eight, she really feels it. Natural exercisers may want to spend more time on physical activity. Foodies may want to spend more time on food. Extroverts may want to spend as much of this time as possible with other people. Your mileage may vary; fine-tune it to fit your individual needs.

If you're thinking, *I can get by with less,* you're right. You can "get by," dragging your increasingly rest-deprived brain and body through your life. And there are periods in your life when adequate rest will not be an option. Newborn baby? No sleep for you. Elderly dog? You'll be up every four hours. Working three jobs while finishing your degree? Get by on five hours of sleep.

But no one who cares about your well-being will expect you to sustain that way of life for an extended period of time. No one in your Bubble of Love wants you to "get by"; they want you to thrive and grow stronger. *We* want you to thrive and grow stronger. What makes you stronger is *rest.*

Suppose you send your ten-year-old child away to camp and you learn they aren't feeding her adequately because they're sure she can "get by" on less.

Suppose you leave your dog with a pet-sitter and learn they're having your dog sleep outside in the cold because he can "get by" in that weather.

Suppose your best friend starts wearing a tight-laced corset everywhere, so that she physically can't take a full breath and is constantly slightly oxygen-deprived, gasping as she climbs a single flight of stairs, but she can "get by" with that much oxygen.

Your child, your dog, and your friend can all "get by" with less than the optimal levels of every basic bodily need. So can you. But the way you react to your hungry child, your shivering dog, and your gasping friend is how we feel about you "getting by" with too little rest. It's not just that we believe you deserve more; it's that we know you're suffering, and we want to bring you relief.

*Sophie worked in one of those high-powered professions where people tend to burn out after one year because the expectation is you'll work sixteen hours a day, at least six days a week. People who stop working at that pace are viewed as failures—they "couldn't take it." They were "weak."*

*Sophie—so used to being both the smartest person in the room and the person viewed as the least valuable—tried to play the game for a long time, but when it didn't work out, she turned to the science to find out why.*

*"Look," she said to her supervisor from behind a stack of research articles, "it says here that people are more creative, more productive, more accurate, and generally do more and better work when they work fewer hours. It seems counterintuitive, but it's true."*

*He didn't believe her and—worse, in Sophie's opinion, because he was supposed to be a scientist and therefore persuadable by evidence—he didn't even read the stack of research.*

*Sophie was learning to love herself more and more, better and better, as she deepened her connection with Bernard. She wanted her work to not make her so, so, so tired. She tried a few other approaches to changing her workplace culture around overwork. She shared a TED Talk about sleep with a few colleagues she liked. She prompted HR to bring in a sleep expert to talk about the neuroscience of sleep and innovation. She changed her own work habits, based on the research, and experienced a boost in creativity and energy.*

*We want to say that Sophie successfully changed the culture of her workplace. She didn't.*

*Instead, she took that boost in creativity and energy and used it to start her own business.*

*She works a lot of hours, but when her body and brain tell her they're done for the day, she listens.*

*"I don't want a doctor who's been awake for twenty hours; I don't want a lawyer who bills more than twelve hours a day—I know how sloppy work gets when somebody is fatigued—and you shouldn't want an engineer who isn't sleeping seven hours a night. Your work is crap if your brain isn't rested."*

## Where Can You Find the Time?

If you're working multiple jobs just to keep a roof over your head and/or raising young children with no help, then you truly might not have ten hours per day to recharge yourself. But let's look at a typical American woman's week, assuming she has a full-time job, a spouse, and two young kids. If your schedule is like hers, then you have time.[36]

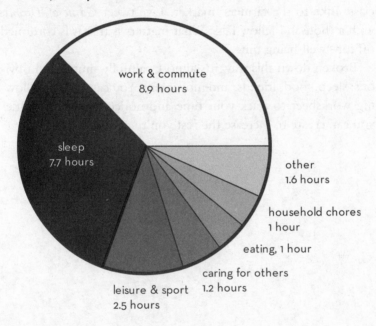

On an average weekday, she spends about nine hours on work—that's eight hours at work and about fifty minutes' total commute time.[37] She sleeps about seven and three-quarters hours. She watches two and a half hours of TV.[38] She spends between one and three hours caring for others, about an hour on household chores, and an hour eating and drinking. She spends her remaining hour and a half on "other"—community and religious activities, shopping, going to school, and grooming.

Boom. Twenty-four hours.

The obvious necessary shifts—more sleep, more exercise—have an equally obvious solution: less time watching TV or shopping or doing chores, whichever contributes least to your "default mode" time.

Sleep is the one behavior that doesn't really allow you to do other things at the same time. The rest of the 42 percent you can use for multiple wellness purposes simultaneously: Connect with your family and friends over a meal or on a walk or at an exercise class. Bike to the farmers' market. Live-tweet *Game of Thrones* with a thousand fellow fans. What matters is that it is cordoned off for "well-being time."

Broken down this way, it's almost painfully simple and obvious: sleep, food, friends, and movement. You can use the following worksheet to track your time and notice the opportunities you can create to increase the rest you're getting.

## 24/7 WORKSHEET

On the first calendar, mark your actual time use. If you have a pretty stable schedule, you can fill it out all at once. If your schedule tends to change, fill it out each day to see how these next seven days go.

1. Block out time for sleep. *At minimum,* it should be a realistic representation of when you really do sleep. Be sure to include in your sleep time the time it takes you to fall asleep and the time between when your alarm goes off and when you actually get up. This is your complete "sleep opportunity."

2. Block out regularly occurring events, including:

   a. work (with commute);
   b. kids' activities and care;
   c. social activities, including those with partner (don't forget sex);
   d. meals, including preparation time;
   e. bathing/showering/hair time;
   f. shopping (including groceries and online shopping); and
   g. TV, Internet/social-media use, solo games, and staring at your phone.

3. Approximate less-regular but anticipatable activities, like doctors' appointments, car maintenance, home repair, etc. An easy way to get a rough estimate is to look at how much time you've spent on these things over the previous twelve months. Add up all that time, divide it by fifty-two, and you'll have the average time per week.

4. Color-code each activity by types of needs they fulfill: connection, rest (both sleep and mind-wandering), meaning, and completing the cycle.

On the second calendar ("Ideal" 24/7 Calendar), imagine the ways you might, hypothetically, make your time use more like the "ideal"—"ideal" being entirely subjective. You're the one who knows whether you need more sleep, more stress-cycle completion, more connection, or just more time.

1. Ideally, your sleep schedule is a solid block of the same seven to nine hours every day, including weekends, but you can make up a shortfall with naps or extra sleep on the weekends.

2. Reserve thirty minutes of each day for a "stress-reducing conversation." If your stress-reducing conversation partner is your life partner, you might also add a weekly hour-long "state of the union" conversation. Research recommends these as the standards for sustaining a satisfying relationship.[39]

3. Include thirty to sixty minutes for physical activity three to six days per week, plus any prep/travel time.

4. Code as before—social, rest, meaning, and completing the cycle.

5. Code some activities, like some phone use, shopping, or meal prep that you haven't been using for mind-wandering rest time, and see if you can transition your state of mind from one of fretful worry to calm future-mapping.

6. BONUS: Mark activities that smash patriarchy. Example: If you work in a job where women are underrepresented, all your work and commute time is patriarchy smashin'. If you parent a child with the goal of transmitting positive and inclusive gender norms, that's patriarchy smashin'. If you are a woman of color, a hijabi in the West, not heterosexual or cisgender, or live with a disability, literally every waking moment is patriarchy smashin'.

The payoff of spending more time resting is that during the remaining 58 percent of your life, you're more energized, more focused, more creative, and nicer to be around—not to mention a safer driver, less likely to make mistakes that will cost you later, and more likely to enjoy what you're doing, rather than simply feeling that it's the "right" thing to do.

We know what to do, and we have the time to do it. Simple. Obvious. Easy. Right?

Of course not. If it were simple and obvious and easy, we'd all already be doing it. So what makes this simple, obvious change so difficult for so many people?

In his book *Why We Sleep: Unlocking the Power of Sleep and Dreams*, Matthew Walker describes our cultural neglect of sleep as a "suffocating noose," and insists "a radical shift in our personal, cultural, professional, and societal appreciation of sleep must occur."[40] For instance, we need schools—especially high schools—to open later, which requires that parents have flexibility about their work hours, which requires that employers prioritize workers' ability to meet the demands of family equally with the demands of the organization. That's just one example of the fundamental systemic changes necessary to create a world where we all have the resources to be rested and well. Getting adequate rest will not be easy.

# REAL 24/7 CALENDAR

| | SUNDAY | MONDAY | TUESDAY |
|---|---|---|---|
| 6 A.M. | | | |
| | | | |
| 7 A.M. | | | |
| | | | |
| 8 A.M. | | | |
| | | | |
| 9 A.M. | | | |
| | | | |
| 10 A.M. | | | |
| | | | |
| 11 A.M. | | | |
| | | | |
| NOON | | | |
| | | | |
| 1 P.M. | | | |
| | | | |
| 2 P.M. | | | |
| | | | |
| 3 P.M. | | | |
| | | | |
| 4 P.M. | | | |
| | | | |
| 5 P.M. | | | |
| | | | |
| 6 P.M. | | | |
| | | | |
| 7 P.M. | | | |
| | | | |
| 8 P.M. | | | |
| | | | |
| 9 P.M. | | | |
| | | | |
| 10 P.M. | | | |
| | | | |
| 11 P.M. | | | |
| | | | |
| 12 A.M. | | | |
| | | | |
| 1 A.M. | | | |
| | | | |
| 2 A.M. | | | |
| | | | |
| 3 A.M. | | | |
| | | | |
| 4 A.M. | | | |
| | | | |
| 5 A.M. | | | |
| | | | |

# REAL 24/7 CALENDAR

| | WEDNESDAY | THURSDAY | FRIDAY | SATURDAY |
|---|---|---|---|---|
| 6 A.M. | | | | |
| 7 A.M. | | | | |
| 8 A.M. | | | | |
| 9 A.M. | | | | |
| 10 A.M. | | | | |
| 11 A.M. | | | | |
| NOON | | | | |
| 1 P.M. | | | | |
| 2 P.M. | | | | |
| 3 P.M. | | | | |
| 4 P.M. | | | | |
| 5 P.M. | | | | |
| 6 P.M. | | | | |
| 7 P.M. | | | | |
| 8 P.M. | | | | |
| 9 P.M. | | | | |
| 10 P.M. | | | | |
| 11 P.M. | | | | |
| 12 A.M. | | | | |
| 1 A.M. | | | | |
| 2 A.M. | | | | |
| 3 A.M. | | | | |
| 4 A.M. | | | | |
| 5 A.M. | | | | |

## "IDEAL" 24/7 CALENDAR

| | SUNDAY | MONDAY | TUESDAY |
|---|---|---|---|
| 6 A.M. | | | |
| | | | |
| 7 A.M. | | | |
| | | | |
| 8 A.M. | | | |
| | | | |
| 9 A.M. | | | |
| | | | |
| 10 A.M. | | | |
| | | | |
| 11 A.M. | | | |
| | | | |
| NOON | | | |
| | | | |
| 1 P.M. | | | |
| | | | |
| 2 P.M. | | | |
| | | | |
| 3 P.M. | | | |
| | | | |
| 4 P.M. | | | |
| | | | |
| 5 P.M. | | | |
| | | | |
| 6 P.M. | | | |
| | | | |
| 7 P.M. | | | |
| | | | |
| 8 P.M. | | | |
| | | | |
| 9 P.M. | | | |
| | | | |
| 10 P.M. | | | |
| | | | |
| 11 P.M. | | | |
| | | | |
| 12 A.M. | | | |
| | | | |
| 1 A.M. | | | |
| | | | |
| 2 A.M. | | | |
| | | | |
| 3 A.M. | | | |
| | | | |
| 4 A.M. | | | |
| | | | |
| 5 A.M. | | | |
| | | | |

# "IDEAL" 24/7 CALENDAR

| | WEDNESDAY | THURSDAY | FRIDAY | SATURDAY |
|---|---|---|---|---|
| 6 A.M. | | | | |
| | | | | |
| 7 A.M. | | | | |
| | | | | |
| 8 A.M. | | | | |
| | | | | |
| 9 A.M. | | | | |
| | | | | |
| 10 A.M. | | | | |
| | | | | |
| 11 A.M. | | | | |
| | | | | |
| NOON | | | | |
| | | | | |
| 1 P.M. | | | | |
| | | | | |
| 2 P.M. | | | | |
| | | | | |
| 3 P.M. | | | | |
| | | | | |
| 4 P.M. | | | | |
| | | | | |
| 5 P.M. | | | | |
| | | | | |
| 6 P.M. | | | | |
| | | | | |
| 7 P.M. | | | | |
| | | | | |
| 8 P.M. | | | | |
| | | | | |
| 9 P.M. | | | | |
| | | | | |
| 10 P.M. | | | | |
| | | | | |
| 11 P.M. | | | | |
| | | | | |
| 12 A.M. | | | | |
| | | | | |
| 1 A.M. | | | | |
| | | | | |
| 2 A.M. | | | | |
| | | | | |
| 3 A.M. | | | | |
| | | | | |
| 4 A.M. | | | | |
| | | | | |
| 5 A.M. | | | | |
| | | | | |

After you finish this chapter and make a plan to improve your rest, you're going to find yourself back in a world that is structured in a way that makes prioritizing rest difficult. But the barriers between women and rest are different and perhaps more difficult than those for men. Because: Human Giver Syndrome.

## The Slow Leak

Human Giver Syndrome puts up barriers between us and rest. We feel guilty for sleeping. We criticize ourselves for doing what is necessary for our own survival and not doing all the other things we could be doing. To sleep as much as we need is to spend a third of our lives not paying attention to the needs of others, and what good human giver would allow that?

*Judging* your need for rest is a slow leak that drains the effectiveness of the rest you get. At the start of this chapter, we said that rest is what makes you stronger, and we already know Human Giver Syndrome doesn't want you to be stronger.

We want you to be strong, healthy, confident, and joyful, so we want you to turn toward those slow leaks and patch them with kindness and compassion.

"Hey there, resentment," you say. "I get it. It's frustrating to be working hard toward a deadline and have the need for sleep slow down your progress. Being a hominid is a drag sometimes, but it's the only family we've got." (Get it? Hominid? Family?)

Or "Hello, worry. You're here because the things I do really matter to me, and you want to make sure I don't fall short. But you and I both know that if I don't get the rest, I'll do a crappy job at all these things that matter."

And even, "Hi, rage. I know our family raised us to believe we didn't matter unless we were perfect, and perfect means we never stop working, and it's right to be angry that we didn't get the warm, unconditional acceptance every child is born deserving.

Let's treat ourselves as we wanted to be treated, granting ourselves permission to be human."

"Oh, you're well rested?" snarks Human Giver Syndrome. "Good for you. Self-care is *so* important. How nice for you, that you have that kind of time."

What a person with that message is really saying is, "How dare you break the rules and treat yourself as if you *matter*? How dare you respect your body, when I'm not allowed to respect mine? What's the matter with you? *Get back in line*."

When that happens, remind yourself that the comment is coming from someone who is suffering from Human Giver Syndrome, just like the rest of us.

"Good for you . . ." says a passive-aggressive colleague, and you can say, "It *is* good for me," in amazed wonder.

You can say, "I used to think it was selfish to prioritize sleep, but then I realized the opposite was true. The people I love and the work I care about deserve me at my best, not exhausted and cranky and unfocused."

Or "I realized I was treating myself worse than I would ever want to see a friend treating themselves, and then I realized that some part of me really believed I should somehow need less rest than they did. How arrogant, right? Accepting that I need rest was a humbling experience, but a necessary one."

Or simply smile. Remind yourself that they're sufffering from Human Giver Syndrome, which is exhausting. You know it is, because you are, too.

## You Can't Spell "Resist" Without "Rest"

Most of the books and articles about prioritizing sleep and rest make the argument that we're more *productive* when we get adequate rest.[41] It's true that rest makes us more productive, ultimately, and if that's an argument that helps you persuade your boss to give you more flexibility, awesome. But we think rest matters not because it makes you more productive, but because it makes you happier and healthier, less grumpy, and more creative. We think rest matters because *you* matter. You are not here to be "productive." You are here to be *you*, to engage with your Something Larger, to move through the world with confidence and joy. And to do that, you require rest.

Our culture treats you as if "being productive" is the most important measure of your worth, as if you are a consumable good. You are a tube of toothpaste to be squeezed relentlessly until empty. For some people and for some parts of our history, this has been explicit and literal, as in slavery. Artist, social justice activist, and founder of Love Gangster Ministries, Tricia Hersey, has established the "Nap Ministry," organizing "collective napping installations" where people of color sleep in public spaces, as commentary on and action against the generations of labor stolen from black bodies in the United States. Her work is a direct answer to the cultural message that people who give their bodies the rest required to survive are "lazy." Sleep is a racial justice issue as well as a gender issue, a class issue, and a basic public health issue. Sleep can heal more than your body; it can begin to heal cultural wounds.

Sometimes we mistake our guilt about resting as our passionate commitment to the people and ideas we cherish most. But in reality, the status quo thrives in a context where people who want to change the world believe that sleep is a sign of weakness and that rest is the enemy.

The cliché that "we won't rest until . . . !" suggests we *shouldn't* rest until the world is, say, a safe place for everyone. But when we deprive ourselves of our own basic needs as mammals under the misguided apprehension that that's how we show our commitment to an issue or to the people we love, we burn out. And then we drop out. Only by making sure we have as much energy coming in as we have going out can we all stay committed to the people, work, and ideas we love. What we're saying is: An overlooked aspect of being "woke" is getting enough sleep.

*Since Julie could handle it, Jeremy continued to vent about his week in charge of Diana's daily routine. He said, "How can I love her so much and yet want to lock her in her room so I can get a break? It's exhausting."*

*Julie nodded. "I know."*

*He rolled his eyes—at her? at himself?—and slumped in his chair. "I know you know, I'm not saying that, and I'm not saying I didn't know. But it's different now. The hard part isn't caring so much all the time; the hard part is sometimes you have to shut off the caring, and it's like shutting off a fire hydrant. I don't want to yell, I don't want to be the asshole dad who yells. I don't want her to think there's anything normal about a man yelling at her, you know?"*

*"I know," Julie repeated, remembering some of why she loved him.*

*"But then she's so infuriating and I want to just— But that's not who I want to be as a father, so I have to swallow it and be calm and not react. I have to enourage her and set time limits and be chipper and explain what's great about doing the thing she doesn't want to do, and it's exhausting," he repeated.*

*"Yeah," Julie said, wondering if he would recognize that she had been doing all that for him for a decade.*

*"I'm a good dad," Jeremy insisted, apparently trying to remind himself as much as her.*

*Julie took a deep breath and let it out slowly, not letting the wave of emotion stick inside her. "Yes," she said. She hesitated, not wanting to pick a fight, then added, "We're both better parents when we get to take a break sometimes."*

*With a tiny laugh at the happy memory, she mimicked his Flynn Rider "smolder" look at him, then said, "The thing about emotions—what I've learned is, you have to complete the stress response cycle that's activated but un-*

*finished because you were staying in control of it. Then you can move to the next thing."*

*"Yes," Jeremy said. Then he said, "What do you mean, 'complete the cycle'?"*

Speaking at Smith College in January 2017, MSNBC host Rachel Maddow answered a question from the audience (full disclosure: from Emily) about how she deals with burnout. She said, "I leave [work] and come [home] and spend time outdoors, and I have the world's most perfect family and great dogs and I go fishing and I chop wood and I use different parts of my brain. And that's the only cure that I really know of; when you are burned out, it's because you burned a specific gear in your brain, but the Lord gave us a lot of different gears. When you use the other ones, you regenerate."

Most of us have spent our whole lives being taught to believe everyone else's opinions about our bodies, rather than to believe what our own bodies are trying to tell us. For some of us, it's been so long since we listened to our bodies, we hardly know how to start understanding what they're trying to tell us, much less how to trust and believe what they're saying. To make matters worse, the more exhausted we are, the noisier the signal is, and the harder it is to hear the message.

Without rest, you are not fully yourself. Without sleep, you will literally die.

And beyond mere survival, rest is a first step to listening to and believing your body.

The next step is learning to live peaceably with that wildly noisy voice in your head that tells you not to rest, tells you you're failing. We call her "the madwoman in the attic," and she's the subject of the next, and last, chapter.

## tl;dr:

- We will literally die without rest. Literally. Finding time for rest is not a #firstworldproblem; it's about *survival.*

- We are not built to persist incessantly, but to oscillate from effort to rest and back again. On average we need to spend 42 percent of our time—ten hours a day—on rest. If we don't take the time to rest, then our bodies will revolt and force us to take the time.

- Human Giver Syndrome tells us it's "self-indulgent" to rest, which makes as much sense as believing it's weak or self-indulgent to breathe.

- Getting the rest your body requires is an act of resistance against the forces that are trying to rig the game and make you helpless. Reclaim rest and you reclaim sovereignty over your own life.

# 8

# GROW MIGHTY

*To understand Sophie, you need to know about the series finale of* Star Trek. *It's called "Turnabout Intruder," and in it we meet Dr. Janice Lester, an ambitious woman driven to madness by her failure to get a captaincy because "the world of starship captains doesn't admit women." Lester forcibly switches bodies with Captain Kirk so that she can finally be a captain, but of course she is foiled, because: Kirk. At the end of the episode, having been forced back into her own body, she sobs, "I'm never going to be the captain," a textbook image of a woman pushed away from her Something Larger, off the Monitor's emotional cliff, into the pit of helpless, hopeless despair.*

*After she's escorted away, Kirk muses, "Her life might have been as rich as any woman's, if only . . . if only."*

*The end of Kirk's thought, we know from things he said earlier in the episode is, "if only she hadn't hated her own womanhood."*

*Sophie's relationship with* Star Trek *became more complicated when she finally got to the end and discovered that's how the whole series ends. It makes Sophie slightly bananas that the series ends with this fatalistic message about the intractability of the patriarchy (ugh), locking women out of the highest leadership positions even in the twenty-third century!*

*Sophie told us, "When I'm doing that progressive-muscle-tension-and-relaxation thing, what I'm imagining is Janice Lester beating the shit out of Kirk. She runs back after that 'if only' comment and is like, 'IF ONLY WHAT, BITCH?! If only I hadn't "hated my own womanhood," you misogynist asshat? I don't hate being a woman, I hate that I only wanted the same thing you wanted, but because of my body, I couldn't have it! And yeah, it made me crazy, and then you said I couldn't have it because I was crazy!' And she beats him to a bloody pulp and everybody's like, 'Yeah, he had that coming a long time.'"*

*The Janice Lester part of Sophie's mind looks at the chasm between reality and hope, and it craves change. Lately, Sophie's been thinking that this part of her might be worth listening to.*

*This chapter is about why that's such an excellent idea.*

Imagine you walk into a room and you hear your best friend in conversation with a stranger.

The stranger is saying, "It's your own fault you got hurt. Why were you so stupid you let that guy near you?"

Or, "Just shut up. Nobody cares. You're not even worth listening to."

Or, "You're a fat, lazy bitch."

How would it feel, to hear this mean stranger say those things to your best friend? Would it be comfortable? Would you ever say these things, in this way, to your best friend?

Of course not.

So why do so many of us say such things to ourselves? Like, every day?

You deserve respect and love; you deserve to be cherished. You deserve kindness, right now, just as you are. Not when you lose ten pounds, or a hundred. Not when you get a promotion or finish your degree or get married or come out or have a baby. Now.

We are surely not the first people to tell you that, and yet the mean stranger in your head is still beating you up. In this chapter, we'll talk about where the mean stranger came from and what you can do about her. As with body acceptance, we can't say you'll end up living a life free of self-criticism. But we can say you'll live a life of more self-kindness, which will lead to greater joy, better health, stronger relationships, and greater capacity to cope when you're struggling.

Let's learn how.

## The Madwoman in the Attic

Amelia's favorite book is *Jane Eyre*. When she first read it as a teenager, she couldn't have articulated the metaphor in the book that so resonated with her: the madwoman living in the attic. Rochester, the hero, has—spoiler—his insane wife locked in his attic. And when you think about it, who doesn't? A demon in our past or our present that taunts us and tries to stop us from doing the things we most want to do. The metaphor is both so ubiquitous and so resonant, whole books have been written about the madwoman as a literary symbol of women's entrap-

ment in dichotomous roles of "demon" and "angel."[1] Activist
and scholar Peggy McIntosh wrote about hers in 1989, describing her madwoman this way:

> *She is alternately off the wall with anger at those who
> have made her feel like a fraud, and off the floor with a
> visionary sense of her own elemental connection with the
> universe. . . . [She writes,] "I MAY NOT KNOW WHO
> I AM BUT YOU SURE AS HELL DON'T, YOU
> GODDOM [sic] PHONIES, SO DON'T YOU TELL
> ME WHO I AM." The other day she looked at me and
> said, "You need me. I'll be here for you." Now, I spend a
> lot of time taking care of her, and when I do it is very
> hard on my family. And here she is telling me I need her.
> Thanks a lot."[2]*

Each person's madwoman is different. For you, maybe she's
more like a shadow, following you around, a perpetual reminder
of what you're not; or a spindly creature lurking under the bed
until you put on some jeans that feel tight or send a text you immediately wish you hadn't sent; or, as one friend of ours put it,
"a whiny, annoying brat of a six-year-old who thinks she knows
everything and will not—give me strength—shut up unless I
take deep breaths for her, then she goes quiet."

Another friend said, "She's the skinnier, younger-looking,
richer, better-dressed, prettier-by-societal-standards, lives-in-the-
amazing-and-much-larger-house-next-door-with-the-perfect-
lawn version of me. On the outside, she really seems to have her
shit together. But I know (and I have to keep reminding myself
*all* of the time) that deep down somewhere in her, she is sadder
and lonelier and doesn't have much more than what is on her
outside, than me."

Still another friend said, "Mine is more like a teenage version:
the smart, quiet, yet sad and downtrodden girl who always sat in

the back of class and no one talked to. . . . When something goes wrong, I can hear her 'told you so' voice in the back of my mind."

Again and again, women describe their madwoman as an uncomfortable, even unpleasant person . . . and they describe her fragility, vulnerability, or sadness.

This uncomfortable, fragile part of ourselves serves a very important function. She grew inside us, to manage the chasm between who we are and who Human Giver Syndrome expects us to be. She is the part of us that has the impossible, tormenting task of bridging the unbridgeable chasm between us and this "expected-us." It's a form of torture, like Sisyphus rolling a rock up a hill only to have it roll back down each time. She's forever oscillating from rage to helpless despair.

If you have beaten yourself up for needing to say no to a friend, that was the madwoman. If you have felt sure that a broken relationship was all your fault, that there had to be something more you could have done, that was the madwoman. If you, like so many women we know, have struggled when you look in a mirror, it's the madwoman you see looking back at you.

When the unbridgeable chasm between us and expected-us looms, our madwoman assesses the situation and decides what the problem is. She has only two options: Is the world a lying asshole, with bogus expectations? Or is there something wrong with *us*?

Some madwomen are more protective than destructive; some are more sad than angry; some have a sense of humor. They are the shadow, the hurt little girl, the downtrodden teenager, the "perfect" version of ourselves, the madwoman in the attic yelling terrible things that echo through the house. What's yours like? Take a few minutes to imagine her—her uncomfortableness and her fragility, both.

### GET TO KNOW YOUR "MADWOMAN"

Describe your madwoman, in words or illustration. Tune in to the difficult, fragile part of yourself that tries to bridge the unbridgeable chasm between you and expected-you. What does she look like? When was she born? What is her history?

What does she say to you? Write out her feelings and thoughts. Notice where she's harshly critical of you, shaming, or perfectionistic. You may even want to mark those places. Highlight them in different colors. Those are sources of exhaustion.

Can you hear sadness or fear under her madness? Ask her what she fears or what she's grieving. Listen to her stories—never forgetting she's a madwoman. Remind her that you are the grown-up, the homeowner, or the teacher, and she can trust you to maintain the attic so that she always has a safe place to stay.

Thank her for the hard work she has done to help you survive.

## Harsh Self-Criticism

In her memoir, *Yes Please*, Amy Poehler describes her madwoman as a demon that "moves its sour mouth up to your ear and reminds you that you are fat and ugly and don't deserve love."[3] (In the audiobook, the demon is voiced by Kathleen Turner.) That is harsh self-criticism, where the gap between you and expected-you is both your fault and a sign of your essential failure in life. The result is guilt and shame.

As Brené Brown says, "Guilt is, 'I made a mistake.' Shame is, 'I am a mistake.'" With guilt, as opposed to shame, there is at least a pretense that one day you might deserve to participate fully in the human experience. With shame, your core self is judged.[4]

Perhaps more insidious than the self-criticism of failure is the self-criticism of success. This self-criticism sneaks in when you win an award or receive a letter of thanks. *"Who do you think you are?"* hisses the madwoman. *"You think you're as good as those other people? Well, you're not! So don't start thinking you might be 'all right just the way you are.' Now,* get back in line!"

## Toxic Perfectionism

Another way that some madwomen wreak havoc is with toxic perfectionism. Perfectionism is a lot of different things—some of them generally benign or even beneficial, and some potentially very toxic.[5]

Generally benign: preferring tidiness and organization over messiness; being detail-oriented and checking your work for mistakes; and having high standards for yourself or others. Any of these factors can become toxic and, at their extreme, are even associated with obsessive-compulsive disorder. That happens when perfectionism functions as a maladaptive strategy to cope with stress, depression, anxiety, loneliness, repressed rage, and helpless despair. But if you're coping well with your feelings (using planful problem-solving and positive reappraisal), then high standards and orderliness aren't going to do you any harm.

Generally toxic: believing that if things aren't perfect, they aren't any good—e.g., if you make one mistake, everything is ruined—and feeling pressure from other people to succeed at everything you do. These domains of perfectionism are associated with depression, anxiety, disordered eating, negative relationships, and feelings of helplessness in the world.

The fundamental problem with perfectionism is that it does terrible things to your Monitor. You have the goal of "perfection," which is an impossible goal, as you start the project or the meal or the outfit or the day, and then as soon as something falls short of "perfect," the whole thing is ruined. And sometimes if your goal is "perfect," some part of you already knows that it's an impossible goal, so you think about your project or meal or outfit or day, knowing you're never going to achieve your goal, and so you feel hopeless before you've even begun.

## Self-Compassion

The opposite of harsh self-criticism and toxic perfectionism is self-compassion. The last twenty years have seen an explosion of research that shows us how much better people do when they engage in less self-criticism and more self-compassion.[6] You've probably heard about self-compassion. You've seen Kristin Neff's TEDx talk or read her or Chris Germer's books or it's one of those things you know you should do, like meditation or mindfulness or gratitude. You've thought to yourself, *Yeah, we should all be gentler with ourselves!* or *I shouldn't be so harsh with myself.*

And you're right; self-compassion is good for you. Or at least, the absence of self-compassion is harmful—it results in self-judgment, isolation, and overidentification with our suffering.[7] Self-compassion reduces depression, anxiety, and disordered eating. It improves overall life satisfaction. When you are gentle with yourself, you grow mighty.

Maybe you tried self-compassion for a while . . . and maybe you slipped back into the habit of beating yourself up.

And then someone reminded you about self-compassion, and you said, "I *know*, I should be nicer to myself; I'm such a—"

STOP RIGHT THERE. That's our sister you're talking about, and we're not going to let you say mean things about her.

If self-compassion is so good for us, why don't we do it?

After a decade of teaching self-compassion and a lifetime of living with our own madwomen, we've found three reasons why this whole self-compassion thing, which seems so appealing, might be surprisingly difficult.

## Self-Compassion Is Hard, Part 1: We Need Our Whips . . . Don't We?

A lot of us spend our lives pushing ourselves to work harder, do more, be better; feeling like a failure when we fall short of someone's expectation; and chastising ourselves for "being arrogant" if we celebrate a success or "settling" if we accept something short of perfection. Often when we experience the chasm between us and expected-us, the madwoman whips us—that is, we whip ourselves. Perversely, we've also spent our lives achieving everything that we've achieved so far, whether that's academic degrees, escaping an unstable family life, attaining financial success, or building a family of our own.

This is the tragedy of the madwoman. She whips us, and we achieve things. And so we think the whipping is *why* we achieved things and we'll never achieve anything without the whipping.

This is the most common reason we hear when people resist self-compassion. They're worried that if they stop beating themselves up, they'll lose all motivation, they'll just sit around watching *Real Housewives* of Anywhere and eating Lucky Charms in a bowl full of Bud Light.

This argument doesn't stand up to even the most superficial investigation. Are we really working toward our goals only because we'll torture ourselves if we stop, so that as soon as we put down the whip we'll sink into eternal apathy? Of course not. In fact, it's the opposite: We only whip ourselves because our goals matter so much that we're willing to suffer this self-inflicted pain if that's what it takes. And we believe that because we've always done it that way, it must be why we've accomplished as much as we have.

Diligent practice of self-compassion works; it lowers stress hormones and improves mood.[8] And many years of research have confirmed that self-forgiveness is associated with greater physical and mental well-being.[9] All without diminishing your motivation to do the things that matter to you.

Many women reading this will find, when they confront their madwoman's harsh criticism and toxic perfectionism, that deep down they know they are doing their best and they can forgive themselves for the ways their best sometimes falls short. They can begin to notice the ways they whip themselves, and practice putting down the whip, because they see that it's not the whip that makes them stronger; it's their persistence, their relationships, their ability to rest. They know that self-kindness helps them grow mightier, and they want that strength.

But for some of us, a harsh, toxic madwoman is telling us we don't *deserve* lower stress or improved mood. She says it's right that we should suffer; we don't deserve kindness or compassion or to grow mighty. And so she will punish us forever, no matter what we achieve.

This dynamic is not just self-criticism, it's self-*persecution*.[10] Folks with more history of abuse and neglect, parental rejection and humiliation are more likely to experience harsh self-criticism and react to it with a sense of helplessness and isolation.[11] When people with depression try to be self-reassuring, their brains respond with threat activation.[12] In fact, fear of compassion *for self* is linked to fear of compassion *from others*. That means that somewhere inside them, they believe that if they're isolated, that's good; isolation protects others from their real, core badness. And if they're suffering, that's good; it prevents them from growing mighty, which might lead to them having power that they would inevitably fail to use effectively, or might even abuse.

If that's you, don't start with self-compassion; start with loving-kindness toward others. *Metta* meditations, as they're known in Buddhism, involve wishing love, compassion, peace, and ease on everyone from the people we care about most to people we hardly know to total strangers to our worst enemies—and even on ourselves. When self-compassion feels out of reach, try loving-kindness for others.

*It was reckoning with her madwoman that finally allowed Julie to feel comfortable with imperfection.*

*Amelia told her about the idea, including the whole Jane Eyre thing, which the English teacher in her loved.*

*"So that's your madwoman?" Julie asked. "Bertha in a back room?"*

*"I think so, yeah," Amelia said. "She's insane and dangerous, but she's also trapped up there by society's ignorance. I have a lot of sympathy for her."*

*"How about Emily? What's her madwoman?"*

*"Have you seen Moana?"*

*"Only about seven hundred times. I have a kid, remember."*

*"Emily says her madwoman is Te Kã, the scary lava monster who, it turns out, is also Te Fiti, the goddess of life."*

*"Huh. It's interesting that neither one is what she appears on the surface," Julie said. "I'm gonna think about this."*

*She did. At first, she thought her madwoman was a "perfect" version of herself. The perfect wife and mother, the perfect teacher, the perfect friend, the perfect daughter. Perfect. Cheerful, patient, wise, effortlessly good at everything, never needing anything. Casually contemptuous of real Julie, with her needs and her flaws and her human limits.*

*Worst of all, Perfect Julie made Julie mean not just to herself but to other people. Sometimes she criticized other people. Sometimes she was mean to Jeremy, for not living up to Perfect Julie's standards.*

*But one Saturday afternoon, she got home from physical therapy to find Diana and Jeremy at the kitchen table together, Diana doing homework, Jeremy grading. Julie looked at her daughter and wondered what kind of madwoman was growing in the young girl's brain, wondered how she was coping with the absurd expectations the world was just beginning to impose on her.*

*And she realized "Perfect Julie" was just a defense she had constructed, to protect her real madwoman—who wasn't a woman at all, but a little girl.*

*This little girl was sensitive and afraid of rejection. She loved books and theater. She put on "Perfect Julie" the way a little girl might put on her mother's shoes and lipstick, playing pretend. She wore "adulting" as a costume. It had been a game at first, like playing house, back when she was Diana's age. But as Julie had gotten older, the Perfect Julie costume became necessary to disguise the fact that she was, underneath it all, just a girl who didn't want to make anyone mad.*

*Once she saw through her madwoman's façade, the rest was easy. From that day on, when she felt the contempt of Perfect Julie, she could turn toward that critical voice as she would to any little girl, hiding behind a mask.*

*"Hey, kiddo," she could tell herself. "You don't have to pretend with me."*

*She could hold the imaginary little girl in her grown-up lap and reassure her that no one was mad and it's okay to need things. People will be there for her.*

## Self-Compassion Is Hard, Part 2: Healing Hurts

For decades, whenever you found yourself falling short of some standard—grades not good enough, face not pretty enough, emotions not controlled enough, loved ones not happy enough—you flayed yourself with the whip, and you worked harder. Each time, the whip opened up wounds in your soul, reopened old wounds, and stung and hurt and made you bleed.

Beating ourselves up results in pain, obviously, so at the same time that we're beating ourselves up, we're looking for ways to manage that pain, to make it bearable. Many of us simply get used to walking around in some degree of pain all the time; we consider it normal. It's the cost of holding on to hope that we will, one day, meet Human Giver Syndrome's standard and finally, at long last, fully belong in the human community and deserve love.

Sometimes the injuries are so severe that we turn to dangerous measures—alcohol and other drugs, self-harm, disordered eating, compulsive behaviors—measures that may numb the pain in the short term, but ultimately deepen the wounds in the long term.

So here we are, telling you to put down the whip.

Reality check: What would actually happen if we put down the whip, stopped beating ourselves up, and turned toward our difficult feelings with kindness and compassion?

Imagine trying it. Let your madwoman put down the whip.

The next thing that happens is that those wounds you've been inflicting and reopening for years . . . finally begin to heal.

And here's a fact about healing that most self-help gurus are not honest about: Healing hurts.

If you break your leg, it hurts. And it keeps hurting until it's not broken anymore. There is no time between the moment your leg breaks and the moment it's healed when it feels better than it did before you broke it. Because healing hurts. And what do you do about a broken leg? You put it in a cast, to create an environment of holding that will allow the leg to heal.

Once you stop reopening wounds you've been inflicting on yourself for years, they finally begin to heal. And it's a *new* kind of pain; it can't be managed by the same strategies you've been using to manage the pain of the whip. You were good at managing that old kind of pain, and now you have to learn a whole new way to deal with this whole new kind of pain. As one client of "compassionate mind therapy" put it, if they started practicing self-compassion, they "would open up a well of unbearable sadness."[13]

A friend of ours, sex therapist Rae McDaniel, talks about this kind of pain as the sting of antiseptic in a wound. It's a healthy kind of pain; it helps the wound to heal cleanly. Reframing it this way (positive reappraisal) helps us tolerate it and helps us find strategies for managing it that aren't numbing or potentially toxic, but facilitate the healing.

Amelia prefers this lobster analogy: A lobster is a squishy animal stuffed inside a hard shell. It grows, but the shell does not. Eventually, it gets too big for the shell, and the discomfort of that confinement leads it to scuttle under a rock, shed the too-small constraint, and grow a new, bigger, thicker shell. The process is uncomfortable, and leaves the lobster temporarily vulnerable, but ultimately it gains new size and strength that it would never have developed if it hadn't gone through the struggle.

Whichever metaphor you prefer, self-compassion isn't always a comfortable or peaceful experience, but it does help us grow mightier. Which brings us to:

## Self-Compassion Is Hard, Part 3:
## Strength Is Scary

Imagine that you've let go of the desire to meet that external standard. You've put down the whip, and those wounds have begun to heal, so you've learned new strategies for managing this new, healing kind of pain.

Then what?

Ah. Then.

As we heal . . . we grow stronger. And stronger. And stronger. Stronger than we've ever been before. Stronger, perhaps, than we ever thought possible. We become strong enough not to feel pushed around by Human Giver Syndrome.

And Human Giver Syndrome will fight back. We will feel backlash. We may fear the world's punishment if we dare to grow mighty.

But sometimes our own strength is scary to us, too. How do *you* feel about the idea of being that strong?

The truth is, a lot of us are scared of how mighty we might grow if we were no longer draining our energy on managing all the self-inflicted pain of self-criticism.

We know that with greater personal power would come greater personal responsibility, and we're afraid when we have the greater power, we won't be able to deal with those greater responsibilities. Let's say you have a hobby that benefits other people, and you start getting paid for it. It turns into a small business, and that small business grows. Eventually, you're going to have to restructure your life, learn about marketing and corporate tax liability, meet with potential partners and clients, hire people and be responsible for their welfare, and now it's not just you and your hobby, it's other people's livelihoods on the line. A lot of us have a quiet little voice worrying that we'll get up in that corporate office and have no idea what we're actually doing. As a person with a hobby, you're not ready for all of that now, and it's difficult to imagine what it will feel like and how ready you could be after you go through the process of growing. The difficulty of imagining ourselves with the knowledge, expertise, and strengths we will gain in the future can stop us entirely from moving toward that future.

Self-compassion: it's hard at first. That's normal. For some people, it stays hard. Also normal. But the result of practicing self-compassion is that you grow mighty. Here's how:

## How to Grow Mighty, Part 1: Befriend Your Madwoman

If you didn't imagine a persona for your "madwoman," take the time to do that. Do it now; we'll wait.

Okay.

The purpose of personifying your madwoman in the attic is to separate yourself from her, to create a dynamic where you can relate to her the way you relate to your friends—with connected knowing. We are, in general, far better at connected knowing with other people than with ourselves.[14] Somehow—and it's not clear why—even the most intuitive connected knower is likely to shift into separate knowing when they relate to their own internal experience. Which is to say, when we think about our lives, we strip our decisions and actions of context and identity; we evaluate them based on the false standards of Human Giver Syndrome. But when we can personify our self-criticism, we can relate to it more effectively. Some form of "personification" appears as a feature of so many different therapeutic modalities, it's clear that many different people and approaches have recognized the power of stepping to one side of our self-criticism and observing it with friendly curiosity.[15]

Personifying our self-criticism allows us to apply connected knowing. With connected knowing, you can separate your *self* from your madwoman and build a relationship with her—maybe even a friendship. This friendship with your own internal experience is powerful. When you're seriously struggling and positive reappraisal isn't enough to make the struggle tolerable, self-compassion can help.[16] In the animated film *Inside Out,* Joy can't cheer up Bing Bong by telling him "Hey, it's gonna be okay. We can fix this!" Positive reappraisal. It doesn't work. Instead, it's when Sadness sits with him and cries with him in compassionate sympathy that Bing Bong feels better. Especially among people with high self-criticism and shame, turning toward your internal experience with kindness and compassion is more healing than positive reappraisal.[17]

There is and always will be a chasm between you and expected-you. What matters is not the size of the chasm or the nature of the chasm or anything else. What matters is how you manage it—which is to say, how you relate to your madwoman.

Turn toward that self-critical part of you with kindness and compassion. Thank her for the hard work she has done to help you survive.

## How to Grow Mighty, Part 2: "Turn and Face the Strange"

That's a lyric from David Bowie's song "Changes." It's about noticing what's happening, no matter what, without actively fighting it. It's really what this book is about: Know what's true. And, if you can, love what's true. But the first step is knowing what's true—all of it. Even the parts that make you uncomfortable. It is perhaps the most potent "active ingredient" in mindfulness.[18]

Sometimes you'll hear this experience described as "acceptance," as in discussions of certain aspects of Buddhist meditation practice. We don't prefer that word, because it carries an unintended connotation of helplessness—as in "Just accept that this is true . . . and therefore abandon any hope that you can change it."

So instead we use the term "observational distance."

Most people are not naturally good at it, but it's a learnable skill.

We'll illustrate this with a comparatively benign example. Homeowners in our part of the world (western Massachusetts) receive monthly letters from the power company, comparing our energy usage to our neighbors'. This kind of peer comparison information has been shown to reduce energy usage, which saves people money and reduces our carbon footprint.[19] In an ideal world, the information would simply remind us to ask ourselves, "Is there more I can be doing?" even if the answer stays, "I'm already doing all I can."

But people *hate* it when the letter says their energy use is higher than their neighbors'. They feel shamed by the utility company; they think the numbers are bogus; they think it's a scam (which is weird—what could the utility company have to gain by making people feel bad for using a lot of their product?). We heard one woman call it "a witch hunt."

So what's going on, to provoke this reaction of shame and rage?

When we're told that our energy usage is higher than our neighbors', the madwoman is activated by the difference between who we are, in terms of our energy usage, and who we are expected to be—super-efficient, yurt-dwelling models of green living. And the madwoman has only two choices: either *we're* wrong or the power company is. Either we're terrible people for burning all that fossil fuel, in which case our madwoman goes on a rampage of shaming self-criticism, or else the power company is a lying asshole for telling us we're burning all that fossil fuel and our madwoman starts ranting and raving about the stupid power company sending us a stupid letter, trying to make us feel bad.

Sometimes the world *is* lying. And sometimes you do fall short of your best.

But when your madwoman flips out in ragey panic, that's your cue to "turn and face the strange." That is, you create observational distance. You calmly and neutrally explore what's actually creating this apparent chasm between you and expected-you. In the case of the power company's letter, what might cause your utility usage to be higher than "average"? Do you live in an old house? Do you work from home, have kids, or charge an electric car? Is your energy use high because you cook at home a lot, which prevents the higher environmental impact of fast-food consumption? Are there a lot of small apartments in your neighborhood, which will definitely require less energy to heat, which will lower the local "average"?

"Is there more I can be doing?" you ask yourself. And maybe the answer is, "I'm already doing all I can," but maybe sometimes the answer is, "I could do a little more." And you don't have to beat yourself up for not having done that little bit more before; before, you were doing all you could. You know that, because you checked in with yourself. You turned and faced the strange.

Everyone's life is different, and we are all doing our best. "Our best" today may not be "the best there is," but it's the best we can do today. Which is strange. And yet true. And could draw us down into helplessness and isolation if we don't stay anchored. And the way we stay anchored is with gratitude.

---

### FACE THE STRANGE, CHANGE THE WORLD

James Baldwin famously said, "Not everything that is faced can be changed. But nothing can be changed until it is faced." Less famously, right before he said that, he said, "And furthermore, you give me a terrifying advantage: You [white people] never had to look at me. I had to look at you. I know more about you than you know about me."

Turning to look at the uncomfortable truths,

turning to face the strange, is the terrifying advantage. People on the receiving end of oppression or violence or the impacts of climate change don't have a choice about it. People with some degree of power, privilege, or opportunity have to *choose* it, the fearful advantage of knowing what is true—all of what is true. Even the parts that highlight the difference between us and expected-us.

The madwoman can't help it. She will flip out whenever she learns about another way in which the world demands more from us than we're giving, and she will try to make it someone's fault—our own or the world's. But look what happens:

Suppose you're a white person, and a person of color points out something you did that was, ya know, kind of racist. Your madwoman flips out, since the world is calling you racist, which is terrible, and you're a good person who would never discriminate against anyone. If your madwoman overreacts and declares the world (that is, the person of color who confronted you) a lying asshole and insists nothing is wrong, then you can't participate in changing the world to make it a better, fairer place. Your reaction is likely to be something like *"That's not what happened! I'm not a racist!"*

If, on the other hand, she overidentifies with the criticism and starts whipping you for being no better than the Klan, calling you a failure and a fraud, then you're too impaired by this self-inflicted suffering to be able to engage productively. Your reaction may be something equally unproductive, like "ALL MY WHITE FEELINGS ARE HURT PLEASE HELP ME BROWN PERSON!"

The madwoman's reactive panic is unhelpful as

a motivation to do anything, but it is great *information*. First, it tells you you're being confronted with a difference between you and expected-you. Second, it tells you that that difference *matters* to you. So an assessment with observational distance might be, "It matters to me that I treat everyone fairly, and it sounds like that's not what happened. I'm always trying to do better."

It's really strange, the experience of "That is not what I meant to do, and yet that is what happened, as far as this new information is concerned." It's really strange when we're doing our best, and our best falls short of what the world expects from us. When we can turn toward that strangeness with observational distance, then we are best enabled to be the change we want to see in the world.

## How to Grow Mighty, Part 3:
## Gratitude (*Sigh*)

It's not a self-help book for women without the injunction to "practice gratitude," right? You already know "gratitude" is good for you. And every time someone reminds you to be grateful, maybe there's a little piece of you that beats yourself up for forgetting to be grateful.

Gratitude practices really are good for you, but before we discuss them, let's mention one caveat: Being grateful for good things doesn't erase the difficult things. Women have spent centuries being told to be grateful for how much better we have it now than we did before. This "gratitude for what you have" has been used as a weapon against us, to silence our struggle and shame us for our suffering. Gratitude is not about ignoring problems. If anything, gratitude works by providing tools for the struggle, for further progress. It is positive reappraisal, concentrated and distilled to its purest essence.[20]

And forgetting to be grateful is completely normal (because: headwinds/tailwinds asymmetry), which is why we all need to be reminded.

So how do we do it?

Gratitude practices as they're generally presented in pop culture—usually some form of grateful-for-what-you-have exercise, like "Every day, write a list of ten things you're grateful for"—don't cut it, empirically speaking. When Emily tried this, it always made her feel worse because it just reminded her of how many people don't have those things, which made her feel helpless and inadequate.

Then she read the research herself and followed the instructions of the evidence-based interventions . . . and it worked like a charm. There are two techniques that really get the job done, and neither involves gratitude-for-what-you-have. The key is practicing gratitude-for-who-you-have and gratitude-for-how-things-happen.

*A Short-Term Quick-Fix Gratitude Boost* is gratitude-for-*who*-you-have. Mr. Rogers, accepting a Lifetime Achievement Award, asked everyone in the audience to take ten seconds to remember some of the people who have "helped you love the good that grows within you, some of those people who have loved us and wanted what was best for us, [. . .] those who have encouraged us to become who we are." That's how to gratitude-for-who-you-have.

If you want to go big, write that person a letter expressing how they helped you.[21] You might even want to give it to them. You might even—and this is only if you want a super-burst of gratitude—read the letter out loud to them. A "gratitude visit" like this can boost your well-being for a full month, or even up to three months.[22]

*A Long-Term Gratitude Lifter* is gratitude-for-how-things-happen. At the end of each day, think of some event or circumstance for which you feel grateful, and write about it:

> 1. Give the event or circumstance a title, like "Finished Writing Chapter 8" or "Made It Through That Meeting Without Crying or Yelling."

> 2. Write down what happened, including details about what anyone involved, including you, did or said.

> 3. Describe how it made you feel at the time, and how you feel now, as you think about it.

> 4. Explain how the event or circumstance came to be. What was the cause? What confluence of circumstances came together to create this moment?

If, as you write, you feel yourself being drawn into negative, critical thoughts and feelings, gently set them to one side and return your attention to the thing you're being grateful for.

The research asks people to do this for three events every day, for at least a week, but Emily couldn't be bothered to do that much, so she did it for just one event per day for three weeks. And it was *great*. It trained her brain to notice not just the positive events themselves, but also the personal strengths she leveraged to create them and the external resources that made it possible.[23]

> *Sophie said to us, "So last night I told Bernard about the mean girls at the department store. And do you know what he said?"*
>
> *"What did he say?"*
>
> *"He put on this serious face and said, 'Your life might have been as rich as any woman's, if only . . . you sweated*

*your butt off on the treadmill and wore a size six.' And I was like, 'Janice Lester!' and he was like, 'That episode is the worst, right?' And . . ."*

*And she kept talking about how the evening went, and it was clear to everyone that she had crossed a threshold. Could there be anything more romantic than a guy who really gets the madwoman in your attic?*

*That was a couple years ago. They bought a house together recently. His kids love her, and she is constantly surprised by how much she loves them. And whenever Sophie encounters what she calls "the usual nonsense," she sends Bernard a text: "JANICE LESTER!!!!!"*

This is the last chapter and the culmination of everything we've learned so far, so let's ask a fundamental question: Why does anything in this book matter? Does it matter how well we are—that is, how free we are to move through the cycles and oscillations of being human? If we're not hurting other people, does it really matter how exhausted, overwhelmed, and self-critical—how burned out—we feel?

It does matter. It matters because we, your authors, want the world to be a better place. We want life to become increasingly good for an increasing number of people. We think you want that, too. And *you are part of the world*.

When you are cruel to yourself, contemptuous and shaming, you only increase the cruelty in the world; when you are kind and compassionate toward yourself, you increase the kindness and compassion in the world. Being compassionate toward yourself—not self-indulgent or self-pitying, but kind—is both the *least* you can do and the *single most important* thing you can do to make the world a better place. Until you are free, we can't be fully free, which is why all of us together have to collaborate to create that freedom for everyone. Our wellness is tied to yours.

The world does not have to change before we turn toward

our internal experience with kindness and compassion. And when we do, that all by itself is a revolution. The world is changed when we change, because we are, each of us—and that includes you— a part of the world. This is our shared home, and we, Emily and Amelia, are your sisters.

## tl;dr:

- We each have a "madwoman" in our psychological attic. She has the impossible job of managing the chasm between what we are and what Human Giver Syndrome has told us to be.

- Self-compassion and gratitude empower us to recognize the difference between who we are and who the world expects us to be, without beating ourselves up or shutting ourselves off from the world.

- Self-compassion is hard because healing hurts and growing stronger can be scary. But it's worth it because healing helps us grow mighty enough to heal Human Giver Syndrome.

- We don't have to wait for the world to change before we begin to heal ourselves and one another.

# CONCLUSION

# JOYFULLY EVER AFTER

We wanted to give *Burnout* an optimistic and empowering "happily ever after" of an ending, but as we finished writing this book, we noticed something strange: our "self-help" book barely mentions happiness.

It turns out we didn't write a book about "happiness."

But there's a different word that appears in every chapter:

Joy.

Isn't joy the same as happiness? Oh, no. As Brittney Cooper writes in *Eloquent Rage*, "Happiness is predicated on 'happenings,' on what's occurring, on whether your life is going right, and whether all is well. Joy arises from an internal clarity about our purpose."[1] When we engage with something larger than ourselves, we make meaning; and when we can resonate, bell-like, with that Something Larger, that's joy. And because our Something Larger is within us, no external circumstances can take away our source of joy, no matter the "happenings" around us.

But it's more than that.

As we considered what it means to live not "happily ever after," but *joyfully* ever after, we realized one last heretical truth: It doesn't come "from within." It comes from connection with fellow givers.

The stepping stone to joy is feeling like you are "enough," and feeling "not enough" is a form of loneliness. We need other people to tell us that we are enough, not because we don't know it already, but because the act of hearing it from someone else— and (equally) the act of taking the time to remind someone else they're enough—is part of what makes us feel we're enough. We give and we receive, and we are made whole.

It is a normal, healthy condition of humanity, to need other people to remind us that we can trust ourselves, that we can be as tender and compassionate with ourselves as we would be, as our best selves, toward any suffering child. To need help feeling "enough" is not a pathology; it is not "neediness." It's as normal as your need to assure the people you love that they can trust themselves, that they can be as tender and compassionate with themselves as you would be with them. And this exchange, this connection, is the springboard from which we launch into a joyful life.

Wellness, once again, is not a state of mind, but a state of action; it is the freedom to move through the cycles of being human, and this ongoing, mutual exchange of support is the essential action of wellness. It is the flow of givers giving *and accepting* support, in all its many forms.

The cure for burnout is not "self-care"; it is all of us caring for one another.

So we'll say it one more time:

Trust your body.

Be kind to yourself.

You are enough, just as you are right now.

Your joy matters.
Please tell everyone you know.

## tl;dr:

- Just because you've dealt with a stressor doesn't mean you've dealt with the stress. And you don't have to wait until all your stressors are dealt with before you deal with your stress. Which is to say, you don't have to wait for the world to be better before you make your life better—and by making your life better, you make the world better.

- Wellness is not a state of being but a state of *action*. It is the freedom to move fluidly through the cyclical, oscillating experiences of being human.

- "Human Giver Syndrome" is the contagious false belief that you have a moral obligation to give every drop of your humanity—your time, attention, energy, love, even your body—in support of others, no matter the cost to you. Pay attention to how different it feels to interact with people who treat you with care and generosity, versus people who treat you as if they are entitled to whatever they want from you.

- Humans are not built to function autonomously; we are built to oscillate from connection to autonomy and back again. Connection—with friends, family, pets, the divine, etc.—is as necessary as food and water.

# ACKNOWLEDGMENTS

Humans are not built to do big things alone; we are built to do them together. Our names are on the cover, but there are scores of humans without whose assistance and support this book wouldn't exist. Here are some of them:

Thanks to our brilliant and delightful literary agent, Lindsay Edgecombe. She sold this book not once but twice, and never wavered in her conviction that a "feminist self-help" book was a great and even necessary idea.

Thanks to our spectacular editor, Sara Weiss, who explained the book to us several times, so that we didn't lose track of our Something Larger, and gave us permission to be super-feminist and also feminine.

Thanks to all the women whose lives went into the composite women's stories. We hope we've done you justice. Thanks to all the people who replied to our Facebook questions. You proved that it's possible to have a substantive, insightful conversation on Facebook—even about intensely emotional topics. Thanks to Charles Carver for writing about the discrepancy-reducing feedback loop, among a great deal else, and for talking to Emily on the phone for an hour. Thanks to Julie Mencher for referring us to *Women's Growth in Connection,* which turned out to be the missing piece of the *Burnout* puzzle.

Thanks to our husbands, without whom we very literally could not have written the book, but more specifically, thanks to Emily's husband for the illustrations, and to Amelia's husband for the music in the audiobook.

We started writing *Burnout* in 2015 and finished in 2018. A lot changed over those years, to put it mildly. #Shepersisted was born in that time, as were the Trump presidency and Brexit. Hillary Clinton became the first presidential candidate to apologize for losing an election. "Incel" entered the public vocabulary, while the #MeToo movement became a global conversation. Maxine Waters reclaimed her time, Emma González called BS, and Dr. Christine Blasey Ford explained the impact of trauma on memory to the U.S. Senate judiciary committee.

In short, the world needs a book about women's survival more now than it has in decades. Writing the book helped us through these difficult years. We hope it offers something in return to all these people who enriched this book, our lives, and the world.

# NOTES

## INTRODUCTION

1. Freudenberger, "Staff Burn-Out Syndrome."
2. Hultell, Melin, and Gustavsson, "Getting Personal with Teacher Burnout"; Larrivee, *Cultivating Teacher Renewal.*
3. Watts and Robertson, "Burnout in University Teaching Staff"; Cardozo, Crawford, et al., "Psychological Distress, Depression."
4. Blanchard, Truchot, et al., "Prevalence and Causes of Burnout"; Imo, "Burnout and Psychiatric Morbidity Among Doctors"; Adriaenssens, De Gucht, and Maes, "Determinants and Prevalence of Burnout in Emergency Nurses"; Moradi, Baradaran, et al., "Prevalence of Burnout in Residents of Obstetrics and Gynecology"; Shanafelt, Boone, et al., "Burnout and Satisfaction Among US Physicians." Another meta-analysis found a range of burnout among ICU professionals between 0 and 70 percent. Van Mol, Kompanje, et al., "Prevalence of Compassion Fatigue Among Healthcare Professionals."
5. Roskam, Raes, and Mikolajczak, "Exhausted Parents."

6.  Purvanova and Muros, "Gender Differences in Burnout."

7.  I.e., women, but also all femmes and people of color.

8.  Manne, *Down Girl.*

9.  Manne, *Down Girl,* 49.

10. Patashnik, Gerber, and Dowling, *Unhealthy Politics.*

11. Friedman and Förster, "Effects of Motivational Cues."

## CHAPTER 1: COMPLETE THE CYCLE

1.  Hippos kill five times as many people as lions—about five hundred people a year—but that's nothing compared to humans; we kill a hundred times that many people in a year. Gates, "Deadliest Animal in the World."

2.  Especially "heart rate variability" (HRV), a measure of how adaptive the cardiovascular system is in response to changes in stressors. Regarding acute stress: Castaldo, Melillo, et al., "Acute Mental Stress Assessment." And regarding chronic stress: Verkuil, Brosschot, et al., "Prolonged Non-Metabolic Heart Rate Variability Reduction."

3.  For example, Marsland, Walsh, et al., "Effects of Acute Psychological Stress"; Valkanova, Ebmeier, and Allan, "CRP, IL-6 and Depression"; Morey, Boggero, et al., "Current Directions in Stress"; and Song, Fang, et al., "Association of Stress-Related Disorders."

4.  Sapolsky, *Why Zebras Don't.*

5.  Similar but not identical—e.g., brain activation varies depending on the nature of the stressors. Psychosocial stressors activate brain areas associated with emotion regulation more than physiological stressors, while physiological stressors activate motor processing more than psychosocial stressors do. Kogler, Müller, et al., "Psychosocial Versus Physiological Stress."

6.  Sofi, Valecchi, et al., "Physical Activity"; Rosenbaum, Tiedemann, et al., "Physical Activity Interventions"; Samitz, Egger, and Zwahlen, "Domains of Physical Activity."

7.  Epley and Schroeder, "Mistakenly Seeking Solitude."

8.  Sandstrom and Dunn, "Social Interactions and Well-Being."

9.  Bazzini, Stack, et al., "Effect of Reminiscing About Laughter."

10. Scott, "Why We Laugh."

11. Grewen, Anderson, et al., "Warm Partner Contact."

12. Walsh, "Human-Animal Bonds I."

13. Christian, Westgarth, et al., "Dog Ownership and Physical Activity"; Richards, Ogata, and Cheng, "Evaluation of the Dogs"; and Keat, Subramaniam, et al., "Review on Benefits of Owning Companion Dogs."

14. Delle Fave, Brdar, et al., "Religion, Spirituality, and Well-Being."

15. Conner, DeYoung, and Silvia, "Everyday Creative Activity."

16. Amy Speace, a singer-songwriter who works with Bessel van der Kolk.

17. Science proves what mothers know: sighing is a sign of relaxation at the neurological level. Li et al., "Peptidergic Control Circuit."

## CHAPTER 2: #PERSIST

1. Aldao, Nolen-Hoeksema, and Schweizer, "Emotion-Regulation Strategies."

2. McRae, Kateri, and Mauss, "Increasing Positive Emotion."

3. Witvliet, Hofelich Mohr, et al., "Transforming or Restraining Rumination."

4. We're defining "optimism" and "pessimism" this way, as a blend of several ways of defining and assessing them. Typical examples include Seligman's "explanatory style," that is, a way of understanding why things happen in terms of the permanence, pervasiveness, and personalness of the factors that cause them. Seligman, *Learned Optimism*. By contrast, Scheier and Carver's Life Orientation Test (LOT) assesses a person's general expectancy of good things or bad things happening. Scheier and Carver, "Optimism, Coping, and Health."

5. Diemand-Yauman, Oppenheimer, and Vaughan, "Fortune Favors the Bold."

6. Mehta, Zhu, and Cheema, "Is Noise Always Bad?"

7. Phillips, "How Diversity Works"; Apfelbaum, Phillips, and Richeson, "Rethinking the Baseline."

8. It's called the "Dunning Kruger Effect." Sapolsky, *Behave*, chap. 2.

9. Byron, Khazanchi, and Nazarian, "Relationship Between Stressors and Creativity."

10. Phillips, Liljenquist, and Neale, "Is the Pain Worth the Gain?"

11. McCrea, Liberman, et al., "Construal Level and Procrastination."

12. Cerasoli, Nicklin, and Ford, "Intrinsic Motivation and Extrinsic Incentives."

13. Torre and Lieberman, "Putting Feelings into Words"; and Fan, Varamesh, et al., "Does Putting Your Emotions into Words."

14. Adams, Watson, et al., "Neuroethology of Decision-Making."

15. Sharp, John, "Senate Democrats Read."

16. Withers, Rachel, "8 Women Who Were Warned; Hatch, "13 Iconic Women Who"; Higgins,"The 35 Best 'Nevertheless.'"

17. Resources for those looking to dive more deeply into the research on what we call "the Monitor" but is technically known as the discrepancy-reducing (or -increasing) feedback loop and criterion velocity: Carver and Scheier, "Feedback Processes in the Simultaneous Regulation of Action and Effect." If you'd like to know more about evidence-based strategies for supporting behavior change, check out Miller and Rollnick, *Motivational Interviewing*. And if you'd like to read the biological and computational science of the "exploit/explore problem," we really valued Ejova, Navarro, and Perfors, "When to Walk Away," and, more peripherally, MacLean, Hare, et al., "Evolution of Self-Control."

## CHAPTER 3: MEANING

1. A review of all survey instruments and questionnaires that scientists and clinicians use to assess "meaning in life" concluded that meaning is "a highly individual perception, understanding[,] or belief about one's own life and activities and the value and importance ascribed to them." Brandstätter, Baumann, et al., "Systematic Review of Meaning."

2. Seligman, *Learned Optimism*.

3. Russo-Netzer, Schulenberg, and Batthyany, "Clinical Perspectives on Meaning." Two-thirds of the studies done in a systematic review of research on personal recovery from mental illness found that "meaning in life" was a significant factor in recovery. Other crucial factors: connectedness, hope, identity, and empowerment, giving the acronym CHIME. Leamy, Bird, et al., "Conceptual Framework for Personal Recovery."

4. Metz, Thaddeus, "The Meaning of Life."

5. Ryan and Deci, "On Happiness and Human Potential."

6. Metz, Thaddeus, "The Meaning of Life."

7. King, Hicks, et al., "Positive Affect and the Experience."

8. Steger, "Experiencing Meaning in Life."

9. Roepke, Jayawickreme, and Riffle, "Meaning and Health"; Czekierda,

Gancarczyk, and Luszczynska, "Associations Between Meaning in Life"; Kim, Strecher, and Ryff, "Purpose in Life and Use."

10. Roepke, Jayawickreme, and Riffle, "Meaning and Health."

11. Vos, "Working with Meaning in Life."

12. Guerrero-Torrelles, Monforte-Royo, et al., "Understanding Meaning in Life Interventions."

13. Park, "Meaning Making Model."

14. "Meaning is knowing what your highest strengths are—and deploying those in the service of something you believe is larger than you are." "Meaning of Life," Positive Psychology Foundation.

15. These are condensed from the Personal Meaning Profile's seven factors of meaning—relationship, intimacy, religion, achievement, self-transcendence, self-acceptance, and fair treatment—and on the Meaning Making Model's self-esteem, affiliation, certainty, and symbolic immortality. Heine, Proulx, and Vohs, "Meaning Maintenance Model."

16. Of course, there are better and worse Something Largers in terms of their impact on the world—to pick the low-hanging fruit of examples, Nazis had plenty of meaning in their lives, murdering millions of people—but the nature of good and evil is outside the scope of this book. If you're asking yourself whether your Something Larger is a good one, consider what our own grandmother told us, which is also what pretty much any major religious figurehead would say: "Ask yourself, 'Are you hurting anyone? Are you helping anyone?'"

17. Hart, *The Ear of the Heart*, 241.

18. Paul and Wong, "Meaning Centered Positive Group Intervention."

19. *Cancer Journals*.

20. Clinton, Hillary, Twitter post, September 6, 2016, 4:18 P.M. https://twitter.com/hillaryclinton/status/774024262352941057.

21. Murdock, "The Heroine's Journey."

22. Friedan, "Up from the Kitchen Floor."

23. Martin, "*Star Trek*'s Uhura Reflects."

24. Park and Baumeister, "Meaning in Life and Adjustment."

25. Tang, Kelley, et al., "Emotions and Meaning in Life."

26. Tsai, El-Gabalawy, et al., "Post-Traumatic Growth Among Veterans."

27. Calhoun, et al., "Relationships between Posttraumatic Growth and Resilience."

28. White, *Maps of Narrative Practice*, and e.g., Vromans and Schweitzer,

"Narrative Therapy for Adults." For depression: Weber, Davis, and McPhie, "Narrative Therapy, Eating Disorders." For disordered eating: Adler, "Living into the Story."

29. Gwozdziewycz and Mehl-Madrona, "Meta-Analysis of Narrative Exposure Therapy."

30. Fisher, *Everlasting Name*. But see also Howe, "I Believe in the Sun," for history and other translations.

## CHAPTER 4: THE GAME IS RIGGED

1. Saha, Eikenburg, et al.,"Repeated Forced Swim Stress."

2. Seligman, *Learned Optimism*.

3. Douthat, "Redistribution of Sex."

4. From July 2016 through August 2018. The Santa Fe, Texas, high school shooting, the Ed's Car Wash shooting, the Marathon Savings Bank shooting, and possibly the Marjory Stoneman Douglas High School shooting were all apparently motivated, at least in part, by jealousy of or rejection by a woman. The Capital Gazette shooting involved the perpetrator's resentment of the newspaper's coverage of his guilty plea to harassment of a woman. Berkowitz, Lu, and Alcantara, "Terrible Numbers That Grow."

5. "Guns and Domestic Violence," Everytown for Gun Safety. Mass shootings are a tiny but highly visible fraction of deaths by gun violence, but they parallel other gun violence, which is disproportionately perpetrated by men and occurs in the context of domestic and intimate partner violence.

6. Krebs, Lindquist, et al., Campus Sexual Assault (CSA) Study.

7. Fulu, Warner, et al., "Why Do Some Men Use Violence Against Women."

8. Sadker and Sadker, *Failing at Fairness*, 269.

9. Karpowitz, Mendelberg, and Shaker, "Gender Inequality in Deliberative Participation."

10. Dalla, Antoniou, et al., "Chronic Mild Stress Impact."

11. Friedan, *Feminine Mystique*.

12. See "Balancing Paid Work, Unpaid Work, and Leisure," OECD.

13. Altintas and Sullivan, "Fifty Years of Change Updated."

14. "Women Shoulder Responsibility," Office for National Statistics.

15. R v R [1992] 1 A.C. 599, House of Lords.

16. Davidai and Gilovich, "Headwinds/Tailwinds Asymmetry."

17. Files, Mayer, et al., "Speaker Introductions at Internal Medicine."

18. "A new study confirms it: You likely experienced that moment of awkwardness or disrespect because you are a woman." Accessed December 7, 2018. https://www.facebook.com/NPR/posts/10155647100291756.

19. Lepore and Revenson, "Relationships Between Posttraumatic Growth."

20. "The Counted: People Killed by Police in the U.S."

21. van Dernoot Lipsky, *Trauma Stewardship*, chap. 4.

22. See Appendix B: Standards of Self-Care Gudelines; Mathieu, *Compassion Fatigue Workbook*.

## CHAPTER 5: THE BIKINI INDUSTRIAL COMPLEX

1. Dohnt and Tiggemann, "Body Image Concerns."

2. Evans, Tovée, et al., "Body Dissatisfaction and Disordered Eating Attitudes."

3. Vander Wal, "Unhealthy Weight Control Behaviors."

4. Becker, "Television, Disordered Eating, and Young Women."

5. "Thick Dumpling Skin"; Cusio, "'Eat Up.'"

6. "Taking Surprising Risks For The Ideal Body." Accessed December 7, 2018. http://www.npr.org/templates/story/story.php?storyId=124700865.

7. Permanent Market Research, "Global Nutrition and Supplements Market."

8. Ernsberger and Koletsky, "Weight Cycling."

9. Risk of all-cause mortality by BMI for women and men, data from *Lancet* table e7 in the supplementary materials, http://www.thelancet.com/cms/attachment/2074019615/2068888322/mmc1.pdf. Unlabeled data points and error values on the graph are as follows:

| | UNDERWEIGHT AVERAGE (ERROR RANGE) | OVERWEIGHT AVERAGE (ERROR RANGE) | OBESITY I AVERAGE (ERROR RANGE) | OBESITY I AVERAGE (ERROR RANGE) | OBESITY III AVERAGE (ERROR RANGE) |
|---|---|---|---|---|---|
| WOMEN | 1.53 (1.45-1.6) | 1.08 (1.06-1.11) | 1.37 (1.37-2.42) | 1.86 (1.77-1.95) | 2.73 (2.55-2.93) |
| MEN | 1.83 (1.66-2.02) | 1.12 (1.09-1.15) | 1.7 (1.62-1.79) | 2.68 (2.53-2.84) | 4.24 (3.77-4.77) |

10. Keith, Fontaine, and Allison, "Mortality Rate and Overweight"; Di Angelantonio, Shilpa, Bhupathiraju, et al., "Body-Mass Index and All-Cause Mortality."

11. Keith, Fontaine, and Allison, "Mortality Rate and Overweight."

12. Park, Wilkens, et al., "Weight Change in Older Adults."

13. Calogero, Tylka, and Mensinger, "Scientific Weightism."

14. Feinman, Pogozelski, et al., "Dietary Carbohydrate Restriction."

15. Schatz and Ornstein, *Athlete*.

16. Collazo-Clavell and Lopez-Jimenez, "Accuracy of Body Mass Index."

17. Saguy, *What's Wrong with Fat?*

18. If you'd like a full account of the political manipulations by the Bikini Industrial Complex that created a world where "healthy weight" means "the lowest weight you can still be healthy" instead of "a wide range indicating general good health," check out Bacon, *Health at Every Size*, or, for nerds, her peer-reviewed academic journal article with Aphramor, "Weight Science."

19. "Why People Hate Tess Munster," Militant Baker.

20. Brown, "These Women Were Fat-Shamed"; Kolata, "Shame of Fat Shaming"; Engber, "Glutton Intolerance"; Chapman, Kaatz, and Carnes, "Physicians and Implicit Bias"; Puhl and Heuer, "Obesity Stigma."

21. Le Grange, Swanson, et al., "Eating Disorder Not Otherwise Specified." "Every 62 minutes at least one person dies as a direct result from an eating disorder." "Eating Disorder Statistics." ANAD.

22. Furnham, Badmin, and Sneade, "Body Image Dissatisfaction"; Kilpatrick, Hebert, and Bartholomew, "College Students' Motivation for Physical Activity."

23. Dittmar, Halliwell, and Ive, "Does Barbie Make Girls Want to Be Thin?"

24. Puhl, Andreyeva, and Brownell, "Perceptions of Weight Discrimination"; Fikkan and Rothblum, "Is Fat a Feminist Issue?"

25. Table 205, "Cumulative Percent Distribution of Population by Height and Sex, 2007 to 2008," https://www2.census.gov/library/publications/2010/compendia/statab/130ed/tables/11s0205.pdf; Lee and Pausé, "Stigma in Practice."

26. Farrell, *Fat Shame*, 145.

27. Ibid.

28. Ibid.

29. Recent examples of this increasingly substantial conclusion: A 2013 meta-analysis found that various diet and exercise regimens could, on average, sustain weight loss of eight pounds over eighteen months: Jo-

hansson, Neovius, and Hemmingsson, "Effects of Anti-Obesity Drugs." A 2014 meta-analysis of the effect of exercise on weight loss found that physical activity sustained weight loss of five pounds over twelve months: Swift, Johannsen, et al., "Role of Exercise and Physical."

30.  For example, the Be Body Positive Model offers five competencies for healing your relationship with your body: (1) *Reclaim health,* by centering your well-being—physical, emotional, social—and shifting "weight" and "body shape" to the periphery. (2) *Practice intuitive self-care,* by listening to your body and attending to your body's need, without trying to control or regulate those needs. (3) *Cultivate self-love,* by practicing self-compassion, or, as Be Body Positive founder Connie Sobczak puts it, "cultivate mercy for your impermanent and ever-changing body." (4) *Declare your own authentic beauty,* by shifting your definition of beauty from the culturally defined standard to "a dynamic, engaged relationship with the world around us." "Declare Your Own Authentic Beauty," TheBodyPositive. You can practice with their online gallery at thisisbeauty .org, where you'll find not just photos, but videos, stories, and poems. And finally, (5) *Build community,* surrounding yourself with people who support you in these ideas. You can read an entire book on the Be Body Positive Model, *embody,* by Connie Sobczak. Health at Every Size (HAES®), similarly, has four principles: Accept your size, trust yourself, adopt healthy lifestyle habits, and embrace size diversity, welcoming the reality that people vary in their size and shape, just as they vary in their race and sexual orientation. "Open to the beauty found across the spectrum," says the HAES manifesto. Bacon, *Health at Every Size,* 274. The Body Project, too, aims to reduce internalization of the "thin ideal" and body self-criticism, and to teach skills of interrupting "fat talk" and "body talk" conversations that reinforce the thin ideal and body self-criticism. Stice and Presnell, *Body Project.*

31.  For a book all about full-on loving your body, see Taylor, *Body Is Not an Apology.*

32.  This sense of your own internal experience is *interoception.* Craig, "How Do You Feel?"

## CHAPTER 6: CONNECT

1. Bakwin, "Loneliness in Infants."
2. Cacioppo and Patrick, *Loneliness,* chap. 6; Gangestad and Grebe, "Hormonal Systems, Human Social Bonding, and Affiliation."
3. Holt-Lunstad, "Social Relationships and Mortality Risk: A Meta-analytic Review."
4. Polack, "New CIGNA Study Reveals Loneliness."
5. Prime Minister's Office. "PM Commits to Government-wide Drive."
6. Hari, Sams, and Nummenmaa, "Attending To and Neglecting People," 20150365.
7. Golland, Arzouan, and Levit-Binnun, "The Mere Co-presence."
8. Cacioppo, Zhou, et al., "You Are in Sync with Me."
9. Goleman, *Social Intelligence,* 4.
10. Gerhardt, *Why Love Matters.*
11. Connection is so fundamental to the nature of being human, so essential to our development, that some scientists argue the socially connected mind is the true "default mode." Hari, Henriksson, et al., "Centrality of Social Interaction."
12. Baumeister and Leary, "Need to Belong"; Malone, Pillow, and Osman, "General Belongingness Scale."
13. Cacioppo and Hawkley, "Loneliness"; Leary, Kelly, et al., "Construct Validity"; Gooding, Winston, et al., "Individual Differences in Hedonic Experience."
14. Nichols and Webster, "Single-Item Need to Belong Scale"; Gardner, Pickett, et al., "On the Outside Looking In"; Kanai, Bahrami, et al., "Brain Structure Links Loneliness"; Beekman, Stock, and Marcus, "Need to Belong, Not Rejection Sensitivity."
15. Robles, Slatcher, et al., "Marital Quality and Health."
16. Coan and Sbarra, "Social Baseline Theory." The authors observe, "To the human brain, social and metabolic resources are treated almost interchangeably."
17. Gottman, *Science of Trust,* chap. 6.
18. Ibid., chap. 10.
19. Robinson, Lopez, et al., "Authenticity, Social Context, and Well-Being."
20. Ibid.
21. Clinchy, "Connected and Separate Knowing."

22. Ryan and David, "Gender Differences in Ways of Knowing."

23. Valdesolo, Ouyang, and DeSteno, "Rhythm of Joint Action."

24. Cirelli, Einarson, and Trainor, "Interpersonal Synchrony Increases."

25. McNeill, *Keeping Together in Time: Dance and Drill in Human History.*

## CHAPTER 7: WHAT MAKES YOU STRONGER

1. Tyler and Burns, "After Depletion."

2. Hagger, Wood, et al., "Ego Depletion and the Strength Model"; Solberg Nes, Ehlers, et al., "Self-regulatory Fatigue, Quality of Life."

3. Tyler and Burns, "After Depletion."

4. Whitfield-Gabrieli and Ford, "Default Mode Network Activity."

5. Domhoff and Fox, "Dreaming and the Default Network."

6. Brodesser-Akner, "Even the World's Top Life."

7. Andrews-Hanna, Smallwood, and Spreng, "Default Network and Self-Generated Thought."

8. Immordino-Yang, Christodoulou, and Singh, "Rest Is Not Idleness."

9. Wilson, Reinhard, et al., "Just Think."

10. Danckert and Merrifield, "Boredom, Sustained Attention."

11. Bailey, *Smart Exercise.*

12. Nowack, "Sleep, Emotional Intelligence."

13. Troxel, "It's More Than Sex"; Troxel, Buysse, et al., "Marital Happiness and Sleep Disturbances."

14. Wilson, Jaremka, et al., "Shortened Sleep Fuels Inflammatory Responses."

15. "Senate Report on CIA Torture: Sleep Deprivation."

16. Everson, Bergmann, and Rechtschaffen, "Sleep Deprivation in the Rat, III." This has never been proven experimentally in humans, for obvious ethical reasons; sleep deprivation is, after all, a form of torture, and has been for centuries. Rejali, *Torture and Democracy.*

17. Itani, Jike, et al., "Short Sleep Duration and Health Outcomes"; de Mello, Narciso, et al., "Sleep Disorders as a Cause."

18. Meng, Zheng, and Hui, "Relationship of Sleep Duration"; Lee, Ng, and Chin, "Impact of Sleep Amount"; Sofi, Cesari, et al., "Insomnia and Risk of Cardiovascular Disease"; Xi, He, et al., "Short Sleep Duration Predicts"; Lin, Chen, et al., "Night-Shift Work Increases Morbidity."

19. Anothaisintawee, Reutrakul, et al., "Sleep Disturbances Compared to Traditional Risk."

20. Kerkhof and Van Dongen, "Effects of Sleep Deprivation"; Fortier-Brochu, Beaulieu-Bonneau, et al., "Insomnia and Daytime Cognitive"; Durmer and Dinges, "Neurocognitive Consequences of Sleep Deprivation"; Ma, Dinges, et al., "How Acute Total Sleep Loss."

21. Williamson and Feyer, "Moderate Sleep Deprivation Produces."

22. Harrison and Horne, "Impact of Sleep Deprivation on Decision"; Barnes and Hollenbeck, "Sleep Deprivation and Decision-Making"; Byrne, Dionisi, et al., "Depleted Leader"; Christian and Ellis, "Examining the Effects of Sleep Deprivation."

23. Baglioni, Battagliese, et al., "Insomnia as a Predictor of Depression"; Sivertsen, Salo, et al., "Bidirectional Association"; Lovato and Gradisar, "Meta-Analysis and Model."

24. Pigeon, Pinquart, and Conner, "Meta-Analysis of Sleep Disturbance."

25. Spiegelhalder, Regen, et al., "Comorbid Sleep Disorders"; Pires, Bezerra, et al., "Effects of Acute Sleep Deprivation."

26. Kessler, "Epidemiology of Women and Depression"; de Girolamo, et al., "Prevalence of Common Mental Disorders in Italy"; Faravelli, et al., "Gender differences in depression and anxiety: the role of age."

27. Liu, Xu, et al., "Sleep Duration and Risk"; Shen, Wu, and Zhang, "Nighttime Sleep Duration"; Cappuccio, D'Elia, et al., "Sleep Duration and All-Cause." There was also around a 30 percent greater risk among those who slept more than nine or ten hours, but many more people are sleeping too little than too much. In one study, 28 percent of American women slept six hours or less, compared with just 9 percent sleeping nine or more hours. Krueger and Friedman, "Sleep Duration in the United States."

28. Fatigue is immensely complicated, from a biological point of view, involving "[a] wide array of immune, inflammatory, oxidative and nitrosative stress (O&NS), bioenergetic, and neurophysiological abnormalities," and hypersomnia can be a symptom of any number of medical issues: Morris, Berk, et al., "Neuro-Immune Pathophysiology." Long sleep is more closely linked to inflammation than short sleep: Irwin, Olmstead, and Carroll, "Sleep Disturbance, Sleep Duration." And long sleep is associated with a 45 percent increase in ten-year risk for stroke: Lee, Ng, and Chin, "Impact of Sleep Amount." It predicts almost all of the health

issues associated with short sleep: Jike, Itani, et al.,"Long Sleep Duration." Seriously, if you're sleeping this much and don't feel rested, talk to a medical provider.

29. Cappuccio, D'Elia, et al., "Sleep Duration and All-Cause."

30. Klug, "Dangerous Doze."

31. Ekirch, "The modernization of western sleep."

32. Hegarty, "Myth of the Eight-Hour."

33. Dzaja, Arber, et al., "Women's Sleep."

34. Burgard, "Needs of Others"; Burgard and Ailshire, "Gender and Time for Sleep."

35. Lane, Liang, et al., "Genome-Wide Association Analyses."

36. People's lives and needs vary, so this is just an illustration. All numbers are from the American Time Use Survey, https://www.bls.gov/tus/.

37. "Average Commute Times," WNYC; McGregor, "Average Work Week."

38. American Time Use Survey, https://www.bls.gov/tus/tables/a1_2015 .pdf. Women in 2015 reported, on average, 0.22 of an hour per day on "participating in sports, exercise, and recreation" and 2.56 hours watching television."

39. Gottman and Silver, *The Seven Principles for Making Marriage Work.*

40. Walker, *Why We Sleep.*

41. Pang, *Rest: Why You Get More Done When You Work Less.*

## CHAPTER 8: GROW MIGHTY

1. Gubar and Gilbert, *The Madwoman in the Attic.*

2. McIntosh, *Feeling Like a Fraud.*

3. Poehler, *Yes Please,* 16.

4. Whelton and Greenberg, "Emotion in Self-Criticism."

5. Stairs, "Clarifying the Construct."

6. Sirois, Kitner, and Hirsch, "Self-Compassion, Affect."

7. MacBeth and Gumley, "Exploring Compassion."

8. Pace, Negi, et al., "Effect of Compassion Meditation."

9. Davis, Ho, et al., "Forgiving the Self"; Macaskill, "Differentiating Dispositional Self-Forgiveness"; da Silva, Witvliet, and Riek, "Self-Forgiveness and Forgiveness-Seeking."

10. Neff and Germer, "Pilot Study."

11. Stuewig and McCloskey, "Relation of Child Maltreatment."

12. Gilbert, McEwan, et al., "Fears of Compassion."

13. Mayhew and Gilbert, "Compassionate Mind Training."

14. Clinchy, "Connected and Separate Knowing."

15. For example: "unblending" in Internal Family Systems: Earley, "Self-Therapy." Or "defusing" in Acceptance and Commitment Therapy: Hayes, Luoma, et al., "Acceptance and Commitment Therapy." Or the "empty chair" strategy of Emotion Focused Therapy: Kannan and Levitt, "Review of Client Self-criticism." It's also similar to "decentering": Fresco, Moore, et al., "Initial Psychometric Properties" and to "self-distancing": Ayduk and Kross, "From a Distance."

16. Diedrich, Grant, et al., "Self-Compassion as an Emotion."

17. Gilbert and Procter, "Compassionate Mind Training"; Gilbert, "Introducing Compassion-Focused Therapy."

18. Gu, Strauss, et al., "How Do Mindfulness-Based Cognitive"; van der Velden, Maj, Kuyken, et al., "Systematic Review of Mechanisms"; Alsubaie, Abbott, et al.,"Mechanisms of Action."

19. Ayres, Raseman, and Shih, "Evidence from Two Large Field Experiments."

20. Lambert, Fincham, and Stillman, "Gratitude and Depressive Symptoms."

21. Toepfer, Cichy, and Peters, "Letters of Gratitude."

22. Gander, Proyer, et al., "Strength-Based Positive Interventions."

23. This is the most effective of the positive psychology interventions. Bolier, Haverman, et al., "Positive Psychology Interventions."

## CONCLUSION: JOYFULLY EVER AFTER

1. Cooper, *Eloquent Rage*, 274.

# REFERENCES

"Average Commute Times." WNYC, n.d., https://project.wnyc.org/commute-times-us/embed.html.

"Balancing Paid Work, Unpaid Work, and Leisure." OECD, n.d., http://www.oecd.org/gender/data/balancingpaidworkunpaidworkandleisure.htm.

"Declare Your Own Authentic Beauty." TheBodyPositive, n.d., http://smedelstein.com/creative/bp/authentic-beauty.htm.

"Eating Disorder Statistics." ANAD, n.d., http://www.anad.org/education-and-awareness/about-eating-disorders/eating-disorders-statistics/.

"Guns and Domestic Violence." Everytown for Gun Safety, n.d., https://everytownresearch.org/wp-content/uploads/2017/01/Guns-and-Domestic-Violence-04.04.18.pdf.

"Relationship Between Posttraumatic Growth and Resilience: Recovery, Resistance, and Reconfiguration." In *Handbook of Posttraumatic Growth: Research and Practice,* ed. Lawrence G. Calhoun and Richard G. Tedeschi. Routledge, 2014.

"Senate Report on CIA Torture: Sleep Deprivation." Human Rights First, n.d., https://www.humanrightsfirst.org/senate-report-cia-torture/sleep-deprivation.

"The Counted: People Killed by Police in the U.S." *Guardian*, n.d., https://www.theguardian.com/us-news/series/counted-us-police-killings.

"The Meaning of Life—The M in PERMA." Positive Psychology Foundation, May 28, 2011, http://www.positivepsyc.com/blog/the-meaning-of-life-the-m-in-perma.

"Thick Dumpling Skin." March 27, 2017, http://www.thickdumplingskin.com.

"Why People Hate Tess Munster (And Other Happy Fat People)." Militant Baker, January 28, 2015, http://www.themilitantbaker.com/2015/01/why-people-hate-tess-munster-and-other.html.

"Women Shoulder the Responsibility of 'Unpaid Work.'" Office for National Statistics (UK), November 10, 2016, https://visual.ons.gov.uk/the-value-of-your-unpaid-work/.

Adams, Geoffrey K., Karli K. Watson, et al. "Neuroethology of Decision-Making." *Current Opinion in Neurobiology* 22, no. 6 (2012): 982–89.

Adler, Jonathan M. "Living into the Story: Agency and Coherence in a Longitudinal Study of Narrative Identity Development and Mental Health over the Course of Psychotherapy." *Journal of Personality and Social Psychology* 102, no. 2 (2012).

Adriaenssens, Jef, Véronique De Gucht, and Stan Maes. "Determinants and Prevalence of Burnout in Emergency Nurses: A Systematic Review of 25 Years of Research." *International Journal of Nursing Studies* 52, no. 2 (2015): 649–61.

Aldao, Amelia, Susan Nolen-Hoeksema, and Susanne Schweizer. "Emotion-Regulation Strategies Across Psychopathology: A Meta-Analytic Review." *Clinical Psychology Review* 30, no. 2 (2010): 217–37.

Alsubaie, Modi, Rebecca Abbott, et al. "Mechanisms of Action in Mindfulness-Based Cognitive Therapy (MBCT) and Mindfulness-Based Stress Reduction (MBSR) in People with Physical and/or Psychological

Conditions: A Systematic Review." *Clinical Psychology Review* 55 (2017): 74–91.

Altintas, Evrim, and Oriel Sullivan. "Fifty Years of Change Updated: Cross-National Gender Convergence in Housework." *Demographic Research* 35 (2016).

American Time Use Survey. "Time Spent in Detailed Primary Activities and Percent of the Civilian Population Engaging in Each Activity, Averages Per Day By Sex, 2015 Annual Averages." Bureau of Labor Statistics, https://www.bls.gov/tus/tables/a1_2015.pdf.

Andrews-Hanna, Jessica R., Jonathan Smallwood, and R. Nathan Spreng. "The Default Network and Self-Generated Thought: Component Processes, Dynamic Control, and Clinical Relevance." *Annals of the New York Academy of Sciences* 1316, no. 1 (2014): 29–52.

Anothaisintawee, Thunyarat, Sirimon Reutrakul, et al. "Sleep Disturbances Compared to Traditional Risk Factors for Diabetes Development: Systematic Review and Meta-Analysis." *Sleep Medicine Reviews* 30 (2016): 11–24.

Apfelbaum, Evan P., Katherine W. Phillips, and Jennifer A. Richeson. "Rethinking the Baseline in Diversity Research: Should We Be Explaining the Effects of Homogeneity?" *Perspectives on Psychological Science* 9, no. 3 (2014): 235–44.

Aphramor, Lucy. "Weight Science: Evaluating the Evidence for a Paradigm Shift." *Nutrition Journal* 10 (2011).

Ayduk, Özlem, and Ethan Kross. "From a Distance: Implications of Spontaneous Self-Distancing for Adaptive Self-Reflection." *Journal of Personality and Social Psychology* 98, no. 5 (2010).

Ayres, Ian, Sophie Raseman, and Alice Shih. "Evidence from Two Large Field Experiments That Peer Comparison Feedback Can Reduce Residential Energy Usage." *Journal of Law, Economics, and Organization* 29 (2009).

Bacon, Linda. *Health at Every Size.* BenBella, 2010.

Baglioni, Chiara, Gemma Battagliese, et al. "Insomnia as a Predictor of Depression: A Meta-Analytic Evaluation of Longitudinal Epidemiological Studies." *Journal of Affective Disorders* 135, no. 1 (2011): 10–19.

Bailey, Covert. *Smart Exercise: Burning Fat, Getting Fit*. Houghton Mifflin, 1994.

Bakwin, Harry. "Loneliness in Infants." *American Journal of Diseases of Children* 63, no. 1 (1942): 30–40.

Barnes, Christopher M., and John R. Hollenbeck. "Sleep Deprivation and Decision-Making Teams: Burning the Midnight Oil or Playing with Fire?" *Academy of Management Review* 34, no. 1 (2009): 56–66.

Baumeister, Roy F., and Mark R. Leary. "The Need to Belong: Desire for Interpersonal Attachments as a Fundamental Human Motivation." *Psychological Bulletin* 117, no. 3 (1995).

Bazzini, D. G., E. R. Stack, et al. "The Effect of Reminiscing About Laughter on Relationship Satisfaction." *Motivation and Emotion* 31 (2007).

Becker, Anne E. "Television, Disordered Eating, and Young Women in Fiji: Negotiating Body Image and Identity During Rapid Social Change." *Culture, Medicine and Psychiatry* 28, no. 4 (2004): 533–59.

Beekman, Janine B., Michelle L. Stock, and Tara Marcus. "Need to Belong, Not Rejection Sensitivity, Moderates Cortisol Response, Self-Reported Stress, and Negative Affect Following Social Exclusion." *Journal of Social Psychology* 156, no. 2 (2016): 131–38.

Berkowitz, Bonnie, Denise Lu, and Chris Alcantara. "The Terrible Numbers That Grow with Each Mass Shooting." *Washington Post,* March 22, 2017.

Blanchard, P., D. Truchot, et al. "Prevalence and Causes of Burnout Amongst Oncology Residents: A Comprehensive Nationwide Cross-Sectional Study." *European Journal of Cancer* 46, no. 15 (2010): 2708–15.

Bolier, Linda, Merel Haverman, et al. "Positive Psychology Interventions: A Meta-Analysis of Randomized Controlled Studies." *BMC Public Health* 13, no. 1 (2013).

Brandstätter, Monika, Urs Baumann, et al. "Systematic Review of Meaning in Life Assessment Instruments." *Psycho-Oncology* 21, no. 10 (2012): 1034–52.

Brodesser-Akner, Taffy. "Even the World's Top Life Coaches Need a Life Coach. Meet Martha Beck." *Bloomberg*, May 18, 2016.

Brown, Harriet. "These Women Were Fat-Shamed by Their Doctors—And It Almost Cost Them Their Lives." *Prevention*, October 29, 2015.

Burgard, Sarah A. "The Needs of Others: Gender and Sleep Interruptions for Caregivers." *Social Forces* 89, no. 4 (2011): 1189–1215.

Burgard, Sarah A., and Jennifer A. Ailshire. "Gender and Time for Sleep Among US Adults." *American Sociological Review* 78, no. 1 (2013): 51–69.

Byrne, Alyson, Angela M. Dionisi, et al. "The Depleted Leader: The Influence of Leaders' Diminished Psychological Resources on Leadership Behaviors." *Leadership Quarterly* 25, no. 2 (2014): 344–57.

Byron, Kristin, Shalini Khazanchi, and Deborah Nazarian. "The Relationship Between Stressors and Creativity: A Meta-Analysis Examining Competing Theoretical Models." *Journal of Applied Psychology* 95, no. 1 (2010).

Cacioppo, J. T., and L. C. Hawkley. "Loneliness." in *Handbook of Individual Differences in Social Behavior,* ed. M. R. Leary and R. H. Hoyle. Guilford Press, 2009.

Cacioppo, John T., and William Patrick. *Loneliness: Human Nature and the Need for Social Connection.* Norton, 2008.

Cacioppo, Stephanie, Haotian Zhou, et al. "You Are in Sync with Me: Neural Correlates of Interpersonal Synchrony with a Partner." *Neuroscience* 277 (2014): 842–58.

Calhoun, Lawrence G., and Richard G. Tedeschi, "Relationships between Posttraumatic Growth and Resilience: Recovery, Resistance, and Reconfiguration." *Handbook of Posttraumatic Growth: Research and Practice.*

Calogero, Rachel M., Tracy L. Tylka, and Janell L. Mensinger. "Scientific Weightism: A View of Mainstream Weight Stigma Research Through a Feminist Lens." In *Feminist Perspectives on Building a Better Psychological Science of Gender,* ed. T. A. Roberts, N. Curtin, et al. Springer International Publishing, 2016.

*Cancer Journals: Special Edition*. San Francisco: Aunt Lute Books, 1997.

Cappuccio, Francesco P., Lanfranco D'Elia, et al. "Sleep Duration and All-Cause Mortality: A Systematic Review and Meta-Analysis of Prospective Studies." *Sleep* 33, no. 5 (2010).

Cardozo, Barbara Lopes, Carol Gotway Crawford, et al. "Psychological Distress, Depression, Anxiety, and Burnout Among International Humanitarian Aid Workers: A Longitudinal Study." *PLOS One* 7, no. 9 (2012).

Carver, Charles S., and Michael F. Scheier. "Feedback Processes in the Simultaneous Regulation of Action and Affect." *Handbook of Motivation Science*, ed. Guilford Press, 2008.

Castaldo, Rossana, Paolo Melillo, et al. "Acute Mental Stress Assessment via Short Term HRV Analysis in Healthy Adults: A Systematic Review with Meta-Analysis." *Biomedical Signal Processing and Control* 18 (2015): 370–77.

Cerasoli, Christopher P., Jessica M. Nicklin, and Michael T. Ford. "Intrinsic Motivation and Extrinsic Incentives Jointly Predict Performance: A 40-Year Meta-Analysis." *Psychological Bulletin* 140, no. 4 (2014).

Chapman, Elizabeth N., Anna Kaatz, and Molly Carnes. "Physicians and Implicit Bias: How Doctors May Unwittingly Perpetuate Health Care Disparities." *Journal of General Internal Medicine* 28, no. 11 (2013): 1504–10.

Christian, Hayley E., Carri Westgarth, et al. "Dog Ownership and Physical Activity: A Review of the Evidence." *Journal of Physical Activity and Health* 10, no. 13 (2013): 750–59.

Christian, Michael S., and Aleksander P. J. Ellis. "Examining the Effects of Sleep Deprivation on Workplace Deviance: A Self-Regulatory Perspective." *Academy of Management Journal* 54, no. 5 (2011): 913–34.

Cirelli, L. K., K. M. Einarson, et al. "Interpersonal Synchrony Increases Prosocial Behavior in Infants." *Developmental Science* 17 (2014): 1003–11.

Clinchy, Blythe McVicker. "Connected and Separate Knowing: Toward a Marriage of True Minds." In *Knowledge, Difference, and Power: Essays Inspired by "Women's Ways of Knowing."* Basic Books, 1996.

Coan, James A., and Davie A. Sbarra. "Social Baseline Theory: The Social Regulation of Risk and Effort." *Current Opinion in Psychology* 1 (2015): 87–91.

Collazo-Clavell, M. L., and F. Lopez-Jimenez. "Accuracy of Body Mass Index to Diagnose Obesity in the US Adult Population." *International Journal of Obesity* 32, no. 6 (2008): 959–66.

Conner, Tamlin S., Colin G. DeYoung, and Paul J. Silvia. "Everyday Creative Activity as a Path to Flourishing." *Journal of Positive Psychology* (2016): 1–9.

Cooper, Brittney. *Eloquent Rage: A Black Feminist Discovers Her Superpower.* St. Martin's Press, 2018.

Craig, Arthur D. "How Do You Feel? Interoception: The Sense of the Physiological Condition of the Body." *Nature Reviews Neuroscience* 3, no. 8 (2002).

Cusio, Carmen. "'Eat Up': How Cultural Messages Can Lead to Eating Disorders." NPR, December 7, 2015.

Czekierda, K., A. Gancarczyk, and A. Luszczynska. "Associations Between Meaning in Life and Health Indicators: A Systematic Review." *European Health Psychologist* 16 Supp. (2014).

da Silva, Sérgio P., Charlotte vanOyen Witvliet, and Blake Riek. "Self-Forgiveness and Forgiveness-Seeking in Response to Rumination: Cardiac and Emotional Responses of Transgressors." *Journal of Positive Psychology* 12, no. 4 (2017): 362–72.

Dalla, C., K. Antoniou, et al. "Chronic Mild Stress Impact: Are Females More Vulnerable?" *Neuroscience* 135, no. 3 (2005): 703–14.

Danckert, Jame, and Colleen Merrifield. "Boredom, Sustained Attention and the Default Mode Network." *Experimental Brain Research* (2016): 1–12.

Davidai, Shai, and Thomas Gilovich. "The Headwinds/Tailwinds Asymmetry: An Availability Bias in Assessments of Barriers and Blessings." *Journal of Personality and Social Psychology* 111, no. 6 (2016).

Davis, Don E., Man Yee Ho, et al. "Forgiving the Self and Physical and Mental Health Correlates: A Meta-Analytic Review." *Journal of Counseling Psychology* 62, no. 2 (2015).

de Girolamo, G., G. Polidori, P. Morosini, et al. "Prevalence of Common Mental Disorders in Italy." *Social Psychiatry and Psychiatric Epidemiology,* 41 (11) (2006): 853–61.

de Mello, Marco Tullio, Veruska Narciso, et al. "Sleep Disorders as a Cause of Motor Vehicle Collisions." *International Journal of Preventive Medicine* 4, no. 3 (2013).

Delle Fave, Antonella, Ingrid Brdar, et al. "Religion, Spirituality, and Well-Being Across Nations: The Eudaemonic and Hedonic Happiness Investigation." In *Well-Being and Cultures.* Springer Netherlands, 2013.

Di Angelantonio, Emanuele Shilpa, N. Bhupathiraju, et al. "Body-Mass Index and All-Cause Mortality: Individual-Participant-Data Meta-Analysis of 239 Prospective Studies in Four Continents." *Lancet* 388, no. 10046 (2016): 776–86.

Diedrich, Alice, Michaela Grant, et al. "Self-Compassion as an Emotion Regulation Strategy in Major Depressive Disorder." *Behaviour Research and Therapy* 58 (July 2014): 43–51.

Diemand-Yauman, Connor, Daniel M. Oppenheimer, and Erikka B. Vaughan. "Fortune Favors the **Bold** (And the *Italicized*): Effects of Disfluency on Educational Outcomes." *Cognition* 118, no. 1 (2011): 111–15.

Dittmar, Helga, Emma Halliwell, and Suzanne Ive. "Does Barbie Make Girls Want to Be Thin? The Effect of Experimental Exposure to Images of Dolls on the Body Image of 5- to 8-Year-Old Girls." *Developmental Psychology* 42, no. 2 (2006).

Dohnt, Hayley K., and Marika Tiggemann. "Body Image Concerns in Young Girls: The Role of Peers and Media Prior to Adolescence." *Journal of Youth and Adolescence* 35, no. 2 (2006): 135–45.

Domhoff, G. William, and Kieran C. R. Fox. "Dreaming and the Default Network: A Review, Synthesis, and Counterintuitive Research Proposal." *Consciousness and Cognition* 33 (2015): 342–53.

Douthat, Ross. "The Redistribution of Sex." *New York Times,* May 2, 2018.

Durmer, Jeffrey S., and David F. Dinges. "Neurocognitive Consequences of Sleep Deprivation." *Seminars in Neurology* 25, no. 01: 117–29.

Dzaja, Andrea, Sara Arber, et al. "Women's Sleep in Health and Disease." *Journal of Psychiatric Research* 39, no. 1 (2005): 55–76.

Earley, Jay. "Self-Therapy: A Step-by-Step Guide to Creating Wholeness and Healing Your Inner Child Using Ifs, a New Cutting-Edge Psycho-therapy." Pattern System Books, 2009.

Ejova, Anastasia, Daniel Navarro, and A. Perfors. "When to Walk Away: The Effect of Variability on Keeping Options Viable." Cognitive Science Society, 2009.

Ekirch, A. Roger. "The modernization of western sleep: Or, does sleep insomnia have a history?" *Past & Present* 226, no. 1 (2015): 149–152.

Engber, Daniel. "Glutton Intolerance: What If a War on Obesity Only Makes the Problem Worse?" *Slate,* October 5, 2009.

Epley, Nicholas, and Juliana Schroeder. "Mistakenly Seeking Solitude." *Journal of Experimental Psychology* 143, no. 5 (2014).

Ernsberger, Paul, and Richard J. Koletsky. "Weight Cycling." *JAMA* 273, no. 13 (1995): 998–99.

Evans, Elizabeth H., Martin J. Tovée, et al. "Body Dissatisfaction and Disordered Eating Attitudes in 7-to-11-Year-Old Girls: Testing a Socio-cultural Model." *Body Image* 10, no. 1 (2013): 8–15.

Everson, Carol A., Bernard M. Bergmann, and Allan Rechtschaffen. "Sleep Deprivation in the Rat, III: Total Sleep Deprivation." *Sleep* 12, no. 1 (1989): 13–21.

Fan, Rui, Ali Varamesh, et al. "Does Putting Your Emotions into Words Make You Feel Better? Measuring the Minute-Scale Dynamics of Emotions from Online Data." arXiv preprint arXiv:1807.09725 (2018).

Farrell, Amy Erdman. *Fat Shame: Stigma and the Fat Body in American Culture*. NYU Press, 2011.

Faravelli, C., M. Alessandra Scarpato, G. Castellini, et al. "Gender differences in depression and anxiety: the role of age." *Psychiatry Research,* (2013): 1301–3.

Feinman, Richard D., Wendy K. Pogozelski, et al. "Dietary Carbohydrate Restriction as the First Approach in Diabetes Management: Critical Review and Evidence Base." *Nutrition* 31, no. 1 (2015): 1–13.

Fikkan, Janna L., and Esther D. Rothblum. "Is Fat a Feminist Issue? Exploring the Gendered Nature of Weight Bias." *Sex Roles* 66, no. 9–10 (2012): 575–92.

Files, Julia A., Anita P. Mayer, et al. "Speaker Introductions at Internal Medicine Grand Rounds: Forms of Address Reveal Gender Bias." *Journal of Women's Health* 26, no. 5 (2017): 413–19.

Fisher, Adam. *An Everlasting Name: A Service for Remembering the Shoah.* Behrman House, 1991.

Fortier-Brochu, Émilie, Simon Beaulieu-Bonneau, et al. "Insomnia and Daytime Cognitive Performance: A Meta-Analysis." *Sleep Medicine Reviews* 16, no. 1 (2012): 83–94.

Fresco, David M., Michael T. Moore, et al. "Initial Psychometric Properties of the Experiences Questionnaire: Validation of a Self-Report Measure of Decentering." *Behavior Therapy* 38, no. 3 (2007): 234–46.

Freudenberger, Herbert J. "The Staff Burn-Out Syndrome in Alternative Institutions." *Psychotherapy Theory Research and Practice* 12 (January 1975): 73–82.

Friedan, Betty. *The Feminine Mystique.* Norton, 1963.

Friedan, Betty. "Up from the Kitchen Floor." *New York Times,* March 4, 1973.

Friedman, Ronald S., and Jens Förster. "Effects of Motivational Cues on Perceptual Asymmetry: Implications for Creativity and Analytical Problem Solving." *Journal of Personality and Social Psychology* 88, no. 2 (2005): 263–75.

Fulu, Emma, Xian Warner, et al. "Why Do Some Men Use Violence Against Women and How Can We Prevent It?" In *Quantitative Findings from the United Nations Multi-Country Study on Men and Violence in Asia and the Pacific.* Bangkok: United Nations Development Programme, 2013.

Furnham, Adrian, Nicola Badmin, and Ian Sneade. "Body Image Dissatisfaction: Gender Differences in Eating Attitudes, Self-Esteem, and Reasons for Exercise." *Journal of Psychology* 136, no. 6 (2002): 581–96.

Gander, Fabian, René T. Proyer, et al. "Strength-Based Positive Interventions: Further Evidence for Their Potential in Enhancing Well-Being and Alleviating Depression." *Journal of Happiness Studies* 14, no. 4 (2013): 1241–59.

Gangestad, Steven W., and Nicholas M. Grebe. "Hormonal Systems, Human Social Bonding, and Affiliation." *Hormones and Behavior* 91 (2017): 122–35.

Gardner, Wendi L., Cynthia L. Pickett, et al. "On the Outside Looking In: Loneliness and Social Monitoring." *Personality and Social Psychology Bulletin* 31, no. 11 (2005): 1549–60.

Gates, Bill. "The Deadliest Animal in the World." *GatesNotes* (blog), April 25, 2014, https://www.gatesnotes.com/Health/Most-Lethal-Animal-Mosquito-Week.

Gerhardt, Sue. *Why Love Matters: How Affection Shapes a Baby's Brain.* Routledge, 2004.

Gilbert, P., K. McEwan, et al. "Fears of Compassion: Development of Three Self-Report Measures." *Psychology and Psychotherapy: Theory, Research and Practice* 84 (2011): 239–55.

Gilbert, Paul. "Introducing Compassion-Focused Therapy." *Advances in Psychiatric Treatment* 15, no. 3 (May 2009): 199–208.

Gilbert, Paul, and Sue Procter. "Compassionate Mind Training for People with High Shame and Self-Criticism: Overview and Pilot Study of a Group Therapy Approach." *Clinical Psychology and Psychotherapy* 13, no. 6 (2006): 353–79.

Goleman, Daniel. *Social Intelligence.* Random House, 2007.

Golland, Yulia, Yossi Arzouan, and Nava Levit-Binnun. "The Mere Co-presence: Synchronization of Autonomic Signals and Emotional Responses Across Co-Present Individuals Not Engaged in Direct Interaction." *PLOS ONE* 10, no. 5 (2015).

Gooding, Diane C., Tina M. Winston, et al. "Individual Differences in Hedonic Experience: Further Evidence for the Construct Validity of the ACIPS." *Psychiatry Research* 229, no. 1 (2015): 524–32.

Gottman, John M. *The Science of Trust: Emotional Attunement for Couples.* Norton, 2011.

Gottman, John, and Nan Silver. *The Seven Principles for Making Marriage Work: A Practical Guide from the Country's Foremost Relationship Expert.* Harmony Books, 2015.

Grewen, K. M., B. J. Anderson, et al. "Warm Partner Contact Is Related to Lower Cardiovascular Reactivity." *Behavioral Medicine* 29 (2003): 123–30.

Gu, Jenny, Clara Strauss, et al. "How Do Mindfulness-Based Cognitive Therapy and Mindfulness-Based Stress Reduction Improve Mental Health and Wellbeing? A Systematic Review and Meta-Analysis of Mediation Studies." *Clinical Psychology Review* 37 (2015): 1–12.

Gubar, Susan, and Sandra Gilbert. *The Madwoman in the Attic.* Yale University Press, 1979.

Guerrero-Torrelles, Mariona, Cristina Monforte-Royo, et al. "Understanding Meaning in Life Interventions in Patients with Advanced Disease: A Systematic Review and Realist Synthesis." *Palliative Medicine* (2017): 0269216316685235.

Gwozdziewycz, Nicolas, and Lewis Mehl-Madrona. "Meta-Analysis of the Use of Narrative Exposure Therapy for the Effects of Trauma Among Refugee Populations." *Permanente Journal* 17, no. 1 (2013): 70–76.

Hagger, Martin S., Chantelle Wood, et al. "Ego Depletion and the Strength Model of Self-Control: A Meta-Analysis." *Psychological Bulletin* 136, no. 4 (2010): 495–525.

Hari, Riitta, Linda Henriksson, et al. "Centrality of Social Interaction in Human Brain Function." *Neuron* 88, no. 1 (2015): 181–93.

Hari, Riitta, Mikko Sams, and Lauri Nummenmaa. "Attending To and Neglecting People: Bridging Neuroscience, Psychology and Sociology." *Philosophical Transactions of the Royal Society B: Biological Sciences* 371 (May 5, 2016): 20150365.

Harrison, Yvonne, and James A. Horne. "The Impact of Sleep Deprivation on Decision Making: A Review." *Journal of Experimental Psychology: Applied* 6, no. 3 (2000): 236–49.

Hart, Dolores. *The Ear of the Heart.* Ignatius Press, 2013.

Hatch, Jenavieve. "13 Iconic Women Who Nevertheless Persisted." *Huffington Post,* February 21, 2017.

Hayes, Steven C., Jason B. Luoma, et al. "Acceptance and Commitment Therapy: Model, Processes and Outcomes." *Behaviour Research and Therapy* 44, no. 1 (2006): 1–25.

Hegarty, Stephanie. "The Myth of the Eight-Hour Sleep." *BBC News Magazine,* February 22, 2012.

Heine, S. J., T. Proulx, and K. D. Vohs. "The Meaning Maintenance Model: On the Coherence of Social Motivations." *Personality and Social Psychology Review* 10 (2006): 88–110.

Herrera, Tim. "Work Less. You'll Get So Much More Done." *New York Times,* June 26, 2017.

Higgins, Marissa. "The 35 Best 'Nevertheless, She Persisted' Tweets, Becaues This Moment Is Nothing Short of Iconic." *Bustle,* February 8, 2017, https://www.bustle.com/p/the-35-best-nevertheless-she-persisted-tweets-because-this-moment-is-nothing-short-of-iconic-36697.

Holt-Lunstad, Julianne, Timothy B. Smith, J. Bradley Layton. "Social Relationships and Mortality Risk: A Meta-Analytic Review." *Public Library of Science Medicine.*

Howe, Everett. "I Believe in the Sun, Part II: The Friend." *Humanist Seminarian,* March 25, 2017, https://humanistseminarian.com/2017/03/25/i-believe-in-the-sun-part-ii-the-friend/.

Hultell, Daniel, Bo Melin, and J. Petter Gustavsson. "Getting Personal with Teacher Burnout: A Longitudinal Study on the Development of Burnout Using a Person-Based Approach." *Teaching and Teacher Education* 32 (2013): 75–86.

Immordino-Yang, Mary Helen, Joanna A. Christodoulou, and Vanessa Singh. "Rest Is Not Idleness: Implications of the Brain's Default Mode for Human Development and Education." *Perspectives on Psychological Science* 7, no. 4 (2012): 352–64.

Imo, Udemezue O. "Burnout and Psychiatric Morbidity Among Doctors in the UK: A Systematic Literature Review of Prevalence and Associated Factors." *BJPsych Bulletin* 41, no. 4 (2017): 197–204.

Irwin, Michael R., Richard Olmstead, and Judith E. Carroll. "Sleep Disturbance, Sleep Duration, and Inflammation: A Systematic Review and Meta-Analysis of Cohort Studies and Experimental Sleep Deprivation." *Biological Psychiatry* 80, no. 1 (2016): 40–52.

Itani, Osamu, Maki Jike, et al. "Short Sleep Duration and Health Outcomes: A Systematic Review, Meta-Analysis, and Meta-Regression." *Sleep Medicine* 32 (2017): 246–56.

Jike, Maki, Osamu Itani, et al. "Long Sleep Duration and Health Outcomes: A Systematic Review, Meta-Analysis and Meta-Regression." *Sleep Medicine Reviews* 39, (2018): 25–36.

Johansson, K., M. Neovius, and E. Hemmingsson. "Effects of Anti-Obesity Drugs, Diet, and Exercise on Weight-Loss Maintenance After a Very-Low-Calorie Diet or Low-Calorie Diet: A Systematic Review and Meta-Analysis of Randomized Controlled Trials." *American Journal of Clinical Nutrition* 99, no. 1 (2014): 14–23.

Kanai, Ryota, Bahador Bahrami, et al. "Brain Structure Links Loneliness to Social Perception." *Current Biology* 22, no. 20 (2012): 1975–79.

Kannan, Divya, and Heidi M. Levitt. "A Review of Client Self-criticism in Psychotherapy." *Journal of Psychotherapy Integration* 23, no. 2 (2013): 166–178.

Karpowitz, Christopher F., Tali Mendelberg, and Lee Shaker. "Gender Inequality in Deliberative Participation." *American Political Science Review,* available on CJO doi:10.1017/S0003055412000329.

Keat, Kung Choon, Ponnusamy Subramaniam, et al. "Review on Benefits of Owning Companion Dogs Among Older Adults." *Mediterranean Journal of Social Sciences* 7, no. 4 (2016): 397–405.

Keith, S. W., K. R. Fontaine, and D. B. Allison. "Mortality Rate and Overweight: Overblown or Underestimated? A Commentary on a Recent Meta-Analysis of the Associations of BMI and Mortality." *Molecular Metabolism* 2, no. 2 (2013): 65–68.

Kerkhof, G. A., and H. P. A. Van Dongen. "Effects of Sleep Deprivation on Cognition." *Human Sleep and Cognition: Basic Research* 185 (2010): 105–129.

Kessler, R. C. "Epidemiology of Women and Depression." *Journal of Affective Disorders* 74(1) (2003): 5–13.

Kilpatrick, Marcus, Edward Hebert, and John Bartholomew. "College Students' Motivation for Physical Activity: Differentiating Men's and Women's Motives for Sport Participation and Exercise." *Journal of American College Health* 54, no. 2 (2005): 87–94.

Kim, Eric S., Victor J. Strecher, and Carol D. Ryff. "Purpose in Life and Use of Preventive Health Care Services." *Proceedings of the National Academy of Sciences* 111, no. 46 (2014): 16331–36.

King, Laura A., Joshua A. Hicks, et al. "Positive Affect and the Experience of Meaning in Life." *Journal of Personality and Social Psychology* 90, no. 1 (2006): 179–196.

Kitchen Sisters. "Taking Surprising Risks for the Ideal Body." NPR, March 22, 2010.

Klug, G. "Dangerous Doze: Sleep and Vulnerability in Medieval German Literature." In *Worlds of Sleep,* ed. L. Brunt and B. Steger. Berlin: Frank & Timme, 2008.

Kogler, Lydia, Veronika I. Müller, et al. "Psychosocial Versus Physiological Stress—Meta-Analyses on Deactivations and Activations of the Neural Correlates of Stress Reactions." *Neuroimage* 119 (2015): 235–51.

Kolata, Gina. "The Shame of Fat Shaming." *New York Times,* October 1, 2016.

Krebs, C., C. Lindquist, et al. The Campus Sexual Assault (CSA) Study (2007), http://www.ncjrs.gov/pdffiles1/nij/grants/221153.pdf.

Krueger, Patrick M., and Elliot M. Friedman. "Sleep Duration in the United States: A Cross-Sectional Population-Based Study." *American Journal of Epidemiology* 169, no. 9 (2009): 1052–63.

Lambert, Nathaniel M., Frank D. Fincham, and Tyler F. Stillman. "Gratitude and Depressive Symptoms: The Role of Positive Reframing and Positive Emotion." *Cognition and Emotion* 26, no. 4 (2012): 615–33.

Lane, Jacqueline M., Jingjing Liang, et al. "Genome-Wide Association Analyses of Sleep Disturbance Traits Identify New Loci and Highlight Shared Genetics with Neuropsychiatric and Metabolic Traits." *Nature Genetics* 49, no. 2 (2017): 274–281.

Larrivee, Barbara. *Cultivating Teacher Renewal: Guarding Against Stress and Burnout.* R&L Education, 2012.

Le Grange, Daniel, Sonja A. Swanson, et al. "Eating Disorder Not Otherwise Specified Presentation in the US Population." *International Journal of Eating Disorders* 45, no. 5 (2012): 711–18.

Leamy, Mary, Victoria Bird, et al. "Conceptual Framework for Personal Recovery in Mental Health: Systematic Review and Narrative Synthesis." *British Journal of Psychiatry* 199, no. 6 (2011): 445–52.

Leary, Mark R., Kristine M. Kelly, et al. "Construct Validity of the Need to Belong Scale: Mapping the Nomological Network." *Journal of Personality Assessment* 95, no. 6 (2013): 610–24.

Lee, Jennifer A., and Cat J. Pausé. "Stigma in Practice: Barriers to Health for Fat Women." *Frontiers in Psychology* 7 (2016): 2063.

Lee, Shaun Wen Huey, Khuen Yen Ng, and Weng Khong Chin. "The Impact of Sleep Amount and Sleep Quality on Glycemic Control in Type 2 Diabetes: A Systematic Review and Meta-Analysis." *Sleep Medicine Reviews* 31 (2017): 91–101.

Lepore, Stephen, and Tracy Revenson. "Relationships Between Posttraumatic Growth and Resilience: Recovery, Resistance, and Reconfiguration." In *Handbook of Posttraumatic Growth: Research and Practice,* ed. Lawrence G. Calhoun and Richard G. Tedeschi. Routledge, 2014.

Li, Peng, et al. "The Peptidergic Control Circuit for Sighing." *Nature* 530 (February 2016): 293–97.

Lin, Xiaoti, Weiyu Chen, et al. "Night-Shift Work Increases Morbidity of Breast Cancer and All-Cause Mortality: A Meta-Analysis of 16 Prospective Cohort Studies." *Sleep Medicine* 16, no. 11 (2015): 1381–87.

Liu, Tong-Zu, Chang Xu, et al. "Sleep Duration and Risk of All-Cause Mortality: A Flexible, Non-Linear, Meta-Regression of 40 Prospective Cohort Studies." *Sleep Medicine Reviews* 32 (2016): 28–36.

Lombrozo, Tania. "Think Your Credentials Are Ignored Because You're A Woman? It Could Be." NPR.org.

Lovato, Nicole, and Michael Gradisar. "A Meta-Analysis and Model of the Relationship Between Sleep and Depression in Adolescents: Recommendations for Future Research and Clinical Practice." *Sleep Medicine Reviews* 18, no. 6 (2014): 521–29.

Ma, Ning, David F. Dinges, et al. "How Acute Total Sleep Loss Affects the Attending Brain: A Meta-Analysis of Neuroimaging Studies." *Sleep* 38, no. 2 (2015): 233–40.

Macaskill, Ann. "Differentiating Dispositional Self-Forgiveness from Other-Forgiveness: Associations with Mental Health and Life Satisfaction." *Journal of Social and Clinical Psychology* 31, no. 1 (2012): 28–50.

MacBeth, Angus, and Andrew Gumley. "Exploring Compassion: A Meta-Analysis of the Association Between Self-Compassion and Psychopathology." *Clinical Psychology Review* 32, no. 6 (2012): 545–52.

MacLean, Evan L., Brian Hare, et al. "The Evolution of Self-Control." *Proceedings of the National Academy of Sciences* 111, no. 20 (2014): E2140–E2148.

Malone, Glenn P., David R. Pillow, and Augustine Osman. "The General Belongingness Scale (GBS): Assessing Achieved Belongingness." *Personality and Individual Differences* 52, no. 3 (2012): 311–16.

Manne, Kate. *Down Girl: The Logic of Misogyny.* Oxford University Press, 2017.

Marsland, Anna L., Catherine Walsh, et al. "The Effects of Acute Psychological Stress on Circulating and Stimulated Inflammatory Markers: A Systematic Review and Meta-Analysis." *Brain, Behavior, and Immunity* 21, no. 7, (2017): 901–912.

Martin, Michel. "Star Trek's Uhura Reflects on MLK Encounter." NPR, January 17, 2011.

Mathieu, Françoise. *The Compassion Fatigue Workbook: Creative Tools for Transforming Compassion Fatigue and Vicarious Traumatization.* Routledge, 2012.

Mayhew, Sophie L., and Paul Gilbert. "Compassionate Mind Training with People Who Hear Malevolent Voices: A Case Series Report." *Clinical Psychology and Psychotherapy* 15, no. 2 (2008): 113–38.

McCrea, Sean M., Nira Liberman, et al. "Construal Level and Procrastination." *Psychological Science* 19, no. 12 (2008): 1308–14.

McGregor, Jena. "The Average Work Week Is Now 47 Hours." *Washington Post*, September 2, 2014.

McIntosh, Peggy. *Feeling Like a Fraud: Part Two.* Stone Center, Wellesley College, 1985.

McNeill, William H., *Keeping Together in Time: Dance and Drill in Human History,* Harvard University Press, 1997.

McRae, Kateri, and Iris B. Mauss. "Increasing Positive Emotion in Negative Contexts: Emotional Consequences, Neural Correlates, and Implications for Resilience." *Positive Neuroscience* (2016): 159–174.

Mehta, Ravi, Rui Juliet Zhu, and Amar Cheema. "Is Noise Always Bad? Exploring the Effects of Ambient Noise on Creative Cognition." *Journal of Consumer Research* 39, no. 4 (2012): 784–99.

Meng, Lin, Yang Zheng, and Rutai Hui. "The Relationship of Sleep Duration and Insomnia to Risk of Hypertension Incidence: A Meta-Analysis of Prospective Cohort Studies." *Hypertension Research* 36, no. 11 (2013): 985.

Metz, Thaddeus. "The Meaning of Life." The Standard Encyclopedia of Philosophy (Summer 2013 Edition), Edward N. Zalta (ed.), https://plato.stanford.edu/archives/sum2013/entries/life-meaning.

Miller, William R., and Stephen Rollnick. *Motivational Interviewing: Helping People Change*. Guilford Press, 2012.

Moradi, Yousef, Hamid Reza Baradaran, et al. "Prevalence of Burnout in Residents of Obstetrics and Gynecology: A Systematic Review and Meta-Analysis." *Medical Journal of the Islamic Republic of Iran* 29, no. 4 (2015): 235.

Morey, Jennifer N., Ian A. Boggero, et al. "Current Directions in Stress and Human Immune Function." *Current Opinion in Psychology* 5 (2015): 13–17.

Morris, Gerwyn, Michael Berk, et al. "The Neuro-Immune Pathophysiology of Central and Peripheral Fatigue in Systemic Immune-Inflammatory and Neuro-Immune Diseases." *Molecular Neurobiology* 53, no. 2 (2016): 1195–1219.

Murdock, Maureen. "The Heroine's Journey." MaureenMurdock.com, n.d., https://www.maureenmurdock.com/articles/articles-the-heroines-journey.

Neff, Kristin D., and Christopher K. Germer. "A Pilot Study and Randomized Controlled Trial of the Mindful Self-Compassion Program." *Journal of Clinical Psychology* 69, no. 1 (2013): 28–44.

Nichols, Austin Lee, and Gregory D. Webster. "The Single-Item Need to Belong Scale." *Personality and Individual Differences* 55, no. 2 (2013): 189–92.

Nowack, Kenneth. "Sleep, Emotional Intelligence, and Interpersonal Effectiveness: Natural Bedfellows." *Consulting Psychology Journal: Practice and Research* 69, no. 2 (2017): 66–79.

Pace, T. W., L. T. Negi, et al. "Effect of Compassion Meditation on Neuroendocrine, Innate Immune and Behavioral Responses to Psychosocial Stress." *Psychoneuroendocrinology* 34 (2009): 87–98.

Pang, Alex. *Rest: Why You Get More Done When You Work Less*. Basic Books, 2016.

Park, Crystal L. "The Meaning Making Model: A Framework for Understanding Meaning, Spirituality, and Stress-Related Growth in

Health Psychology." *European Health Psychologist* 15, no. 2 (2013): 40–47.

Park, Jina, and Roy F. Baumeister. "Meaning in Life and Adjustment to Daily Stressors." *Journal of Positive Psychology* 12, no. 4 (2017): 333–41.

Park, Song-Yi, Lynne R. Wilkens, et al. "Weight Change in Older Adults and Mortality: The Multiethnic Cohort Study." *International Journal of Obesity* 42, no. 2 (2018): 205–212.

Patashnik, Erik M., Alan S. Gerber, and Conor M. Dowling. *Unhealthy Politics: The Battle Over Evidence-Based Medicine*. Princeton University Press, 2017.

Paul, T., and P. Wong. "Meaning Centered Positive Group Intervention." In *Clinical Perspectives on Meaning*. Springer International, 2016.

Permanent Market Research. "Global Nutrition and Supplements Market: History, Industry Growth, and Future Trends by PMR." Globe NewsWire.com, January 27, 2015, https://globenewswire.com/news-release/2015/01/27/700276/10117198/en/Global-Nutrition-and-Supplements-Market-History-Industry-Growth-and-Future-Trends-by-PMR.html.

Phillips, Katherine W. "How Diversity Works." *Scientific American* 311, no. 4 (2014): 42–47.

Phillips, Katherine W., Katie A. Liljenquist, and Margaret A. Neale. "Is the Pain Worth the Gain? The Advantages and Liabilities of Agreeing with Socially Distinct Newcomers." *Personality and Social Psychology Bulletin* 35, no. 3 (2009): 336–50.

Pigeon, Wilfred R., Martin Pinquart, and Kenneth Conner. "Meta-Analysis of Sleep Disturbance and Suicidal Thoughts and Behaviors." *Journal of Clinical Psychiatry* 73, no. 9 (2012): 1160–67.

Pires, Gabriel Natan, Andreia Gomes Bezerra, et al. "Effects of Acute Sleep Deprivation on State Anxiety Levels: A Systematic Review and Meta-Analysis." *Sleep Medicine* 24 (2016): 109–18.

Poehler, Amy. *Yes Please*. Dey Street, 2014.

Polack, Ellie. "New CIGNA Study Reveals Loneliness at Epidemic Levels in America." CIGNA, May 1, 2018, https://www.multivu.com/players/English/8294451-cigna-us-loneliness-survey/docs/IndexReport_15240 69371598–173525450.pdf.

Prime Minister's Office. "PM Commits to Government-wide Drive to Tackle Loneliness," Gov.uk, January 17, 2018, https://www.gov.uk/government/news/pm-commits-to-government-wide-drive-to-tackle -loneliness.

Puhl, Rebecca M., and Chelsea A. Heuer. "Obesity Stigma: Important Considerations for Public Health." *American Journal of Public Health* 100, no. 6 (2010): 1019–28.

Puhl, Rebecca M., Tatiana Andreyeva, and Kelly D. Brownell. "Perceptions of Weight Discrimination: Prevalence and Comparison to Race and Gender Discrimination in America." *International Journal of Obesity* 32, no. 6 (2008): 992–1000.

Purvanova, Radostina K., and John P. Muros. "Gender Differences in Burnout: A Meta-Analysis." *Journal of Vocational Behavior* 77, no. 2 (2010): 168–85.

Rejali, Darius. *Torture and Democracy.* Princeton University Press, 2009.

Richards, Elizabeth A., Niwako Ogata, and Ching-Wei Cheng. "Evaluation of the Dogs, Physical Activity, and Walking (Dogs PAW) Intervention: A Randomized Controlled Trial." *Nursing Research* 65, no. 3 (2016): 191–201.

Robinson, Oliver C., Frederick G. Lopez, et al. "Authenticity, Social Context, and Well-Being in the United States, England, and Russia: A Three Country Comparative Analysis." *Journal of Cross-Cultural Psychology* 44, no. 5 (2013): 719–37.

Robles, Theodore F., Richard B. Slatcher, et al. "Marital Quality and Health: A Meta-Analytic Review." *Psychological Bulletin* 140, no. 1 (2014): 140–187.

Roepke, Ann Marie, Eranda Jayawickreme, and Olivia M. Riffle. "Meaning and Health: A Systematic Review." *Applied Research in Quality of Life* 9, no. 4 (2014): 1055–79.

Rosenbaum, Simon, Anne Tiedemann, Catherine Sherrington, Jackie Curtis, and Philip B. Ward. "Physical Activity Interventions for People with Mental Illness: A Systematic Review and Meta-Analysis." *Journal of Clinical Psychiatry* 75, no. 9 (2014): 964–74.

Roskam, Isabelle, Marie-Emilie Raes, and Moïra Mikolajczak. "Exhausted Parents: Development and Preliminary Validation of the Parental Burnout Inventory." *Frontiers in Psychology* 8 (2017): 163.

Russo-Netzer, Pninit, Stefan E. Schulenberg, and Alexander Batthyany. "Clinical Perspectives on Meaning: Understanding, Coping and Thriving Through Science and Practice." In *Clinical Perspectives on Meaning*. Springer International Publishing, 2016.

Ryan, Michelle K., and Barbara David. "Gender Differences in Ways of Knowing: The Context Dependence of the Attitudes Toward Thinking and Learning Survey." *Sex Roles* 49, no. 11-12 (2003): 693–99.

Ryan, Richard M., and Edward L. Deci. "On Happiness and Human Potentials: A Review of Research on Hedonic and Eudaimonic Well-Being." *Annual Review of Psychology* 52, no. 1 (2001): 141–66.

Sadker, Myra, and David Sadker. *Failing at Fairness: How America's Schools Cheat Girls*. Simon & Schuster, 2010.

Saguy, Abigail C. *What's Wrong with Fat?* Oxford University Press, 2012.

Saha, Kaustuv, Douglas Eikenburg, et al. "Repeated Forced Swim Stress Induces Learned Helplessness in Rats." *FASEB Journal* 26, no. 1 supp. (2012): 1042–48.

Samitz, Guenther, Matthias Egger, and Marcel Zwahlen. "Domains of Physical Activity and All-Cause Mortality: Systematic Review and Dose-Response Meta-Analysis of Cohort Studies." *International Journal of Epidemiology* 40, no. 5 (2011): 1382–1400.

Sandstrom, Gillian M., and Elizabeth W. Dunn. "Social Interactions and Well-Being: The Surprising Power of Weak Ties." *Personality and Social Psychology Bulletin* 40, no. 7 (2014): 910–22.

Sapolsky, Robert. *Behave: The Biology of Humans at Our Best and Worst*. Penguin, 2017.

Sapolsky, Robert. *Why Zebras Don't Get Ulcers*. Holt, 2004.

Schatz, Howard, and Beverly Ornstein. *Athlete*. Harper Collins, 2002.

Scheier, Michael F., and Charles S. Carver. "Optimism, Coping, and Health: Assessment and Implications of Generalized Outcome Expectancies." *Health Psychology* 4, no. 3 (1985): 219.

Scott, Sophie. "Why We Laugh." *TED: Ideas Worth Spreading,* March 2015, https://www.ted.com/talks/sophie_scott_why_we_laugh?language=en.

Seligman, Martin E. P. *Learned Optimism: How to Change Your Mind and Your Life*. Vintage, 2006.

Shanafelt, Tait D., Sonja Boone, et al. "Burnout and Satisfaction with Work-Life Balance Among US Physicians Relative to the General US Population." *Archives of Internal Medicine* 172, no. 18 (2012): 1377–85.

Sharp, John. "Senate Democrats Read Coretta Scott King Letter in Opposition to Jeff Sessions." Alabama.com, February. 8, 2017, https://www.al.com/news/mobile/index.ssf/2017/02/senate_democrats_read_coretta.html.

Shen, Xiaoli, Yili Wu, and Dongfeng Zhang. "Nighttime Sleep Duration, 24-Hour Sleep Duration and Risk of All-Cause Mortality Among Adults: A Meta-Analysis of Prospective Cohort Studies." *Scientific Reports* 6 (2016).

Sirois, Fuschia M., Ryan Kitner, and Jameson K. Hirsch. "Self-compassion, Affect, and Health-Promoting Behaviors." *Health Psychology* 34, no. 6 (2015): 661.

Sivertsen, Børge, Paula Salo, et al. "The Bidirectional Association Between Depression and Insomnia: The HUNT Study." *Psychosomatic Medicine* 74, no. 7 (2012): 758–65.

Sobczak, Connie. *Embody: Learning to Love Your Unique Body* (and quiet that critical voice!). Gurze Books, 2014.

Sofi, Francesco, D. Valecchi, et al. "Physical Activity and Risk of Cognitive Decline: A Meta-Analysis of Prospective Studies." *Journal of Internal Medicine* 269, no. 1 (2011): 107–17.

Sofi, Francesco, Francesca Cesari, et al. "Insomnia and Risk of Cardiovascular Disease: A Meta-Analysis." *European Journal of Preventive Cardiology* 21, no. 1 (2014): 57–64.

Solberg Nes, Lise, Shawna L. Ehlers, et al. "Self-regulatory Fatigue, Quality of Life, Health Behaviors, and Coping in Patients with Hematologic Malignancies." *Annals of Behavioral Medicine* 48, no. 3 (2014): 411–23.

Song, Huan, Fang Fang, et al. "Association of Stress-Related Disorders with Subsequent Autoimmune Disease." *JAMA* 319, no. 23 (2018): 2388–400.

Spiegelhalder, Kai, Wolfram Regen, et al. "Comorbid Sleep Disorders in Neuropsychiatric Disorders Across the Life Cycle." *Current Psychiatry Reports* 15, no. 6 (2013): 1–6.

Stairs, Agnes M., Gregory T. Smith, et al. "Clarifying the Construct of Perfectionism." *Assessment* 19, no. 2 (2012): 146–66.

Steakley, Lia. "Promoting Healthy Eating and a Positive Body Image on College Campuses." *Scope, Stanford Medicine,* May 29, 2014, https://stan.md/2xwwbyw.

Steger, Michael F. "Experiencing Meaning in Life." In *The Human Quest for Meaning: Theories, Research, and Applications.* Routledge, 2012.

Stice, Eric, and Katherine Presnell. *The Body Project: Promoting Body Acceptance and Preventing Eating Disorders.* Oxford University Press, 2007.

Stuewig, J., and L. A. McCloskey. "The Relation of Child Maltreatment to Shame and Guilt Among Adolescents: Psychological Routes to Depression and Deliquency." *Child Maltreatment* 10 (2005): 324–36.

Swift, D. L., N. M. Johannsen, et al. "The Role of Exercise and Physical Activity in Weight Loss and Maintenance." *Progress in Cardiovascular Disease* 56, no. 4 ( 2014): 441–47.

Tang, David, Nicholas J. Kelley, et al. "Emotions and Meaning in Life: A Motivational Perspective." In *The Experience of Meaning in Life.* Springer Netherlands, 2013.

Taylor, Sonya Renee. *The Body Is Not an Apology: The Power of Radical Self-Love*. Berrett-Koehler, 2018.

Toepfer, Steven M., Kelly Cichy, and Patti Peters. "Letters of Gratitude: Further Evidence for Author Benefits." *Journal of Happiness Studies* 13, no. 1 (2012): 187–201.

Torre, Jared B., and Matthew D. Lieberman. "Putting Feelings into Words: Affect Labeling as Implicit Emotion Regulation." *Emotion Review* 10, no. 2 (2018): 116–24.

Troxel, Wendy M. "It's More Than Sex: Exploring the Dyadic Nature of Sleep and Implications for Health." *Psychosomatic Medicine* 72, no. 6 (2010): 578.

Troxel, Wendy M., Daniel J. Buysse, et al. "Marital Happiness and Sleep Disturbances in a Multi-ethnic Sample of Middle-Aged Women." *Behavioral Sleep Medicine* 7, no. 1 (2009): 2–19.

Tsai, J., R. El-Gabalawy, et al. "Post-traumatic Growth Among Veterans in the USA: Results from the National Health and Resilience in Veterans Study." *Psychological Medicine* 45, no. 01 (2015): 165–79.

Tyler, James M., and Kathleen C. Burns. "After Depletion: The Replenishment of the Self's Regulatory Resources." *Self and Identity* 7, no. 3 (2008): 305–21.

Valdesolo, Piercarlo, Jennifer Ouyang, and David De Steno. "The Rhythm of Joint Action: Synchrony Promotes Cooperative Ability." *Journal of Experimental Social Psychology* 46, no. 4 (July 2010): 693–95.

Valkanova, Vyara, Klaus P. Ebmeier, and Charlotte L. Allan. "CRP, IL-6 and Depression: A Systematic Review and Meta-Analysis of Longitudinal Studies." *Journal of Affective Disorders* 150, no. 3 (2013): 736–44.

van der Velden, Anne Maj, Willem Kuyken, et al. "A Systematic Review of Mechanisms of Change in Mindfulness-Based Cognitive Therapy in the Treatment of Recurrent Major Depressive Disorder." *Clinical Psychology Review* 37 (2015): 26–39.

van Dernoot Lipsky, Laura. *Trauma Stewardship: An Everyday Guide to Caring for Self While Caring for Others*. ReadHowYouWant.com, 2010.

van Mol, M. M., E. J. Kompanje, et al. "The Prevalence of Compassion Fatigue and Burnout Among Healthcare Professionals in Intensive Care Units: A Systematic Review." *PLOS One* 10, no. 8 (2015): p. e0136955.

Vander Wal, Jillon S. "Unhealthy Weight Control Behaviors Among Adolescents." *Journal of Health Psychology* 17, no. 1 (2012): 110–20.

Verkuil, Bart, Jos F. Brosschot, et al. "Prolonged Non-Metabolic Heart Rate Variability Reduction as a Physiological Marker of Psychological Stress in Daily Life." *Annals of Behavioral Medicine* 50, no. 5 (2016): 704–14.

Vos, Joel. "Working with Meaning in Life in Mental Health Care: A Systematic Literature Review of the Practices and Effectiveness of Meaning-Centred Therapies." In *Clinical Perspectives on Meaning*, ed. Russo-Netzer P., Schulenberg S., Batthyany A. Springer International, 2016.

Vromans, Lynette P., and Robert D. Schweitzer. "Narrative Therapy for Adults with Major Depressive Disorder: Improved Symptom and Interpersonal Outcomes." *Psychotherapy Research* 21, no. 1 (2011): 4–15.

Walker, Matthew. *Why We Sleep: Unlocking the Power of Sleep and Dreams*. Simon & Schuster, 2017.

Walsh, Froma. "Human-Animal Bonds I: The Relational Significance of Companion Animals." *Family Process* 48, no. 4 (2009): 462–80.

Watts, Jenny, and Noelle Robertson. "Burnout in University Teaching Staff: A Systematic Literature Review." *Educational Research* 53, no. 1 (2011): 33–50.

Weber, Mim, Kierrynn Davis, and Lisa McPhie. "Narrative Therapy, Eating Disorders and Groups: Enhancing Outcomes in Rural NSW." *Australian Social Work* 59, no. 4 (2006): 391–405.

Whelton, William J., and Leslie S. Greenberg. "Emotion in Self-Criticism." *Personality and Individual Differences* 38, no. 7 (2005): 1583–95.

White, Michael. *Maps of Narrative Practice*. Norton, 2007.

Whitfield-Gabrieli, Susan, and Judith M. Ford. "Default Mode Network Activity and Connectivity in Psychopathology." *Annual Review of Clinical Psychology* 8 (2012): 49–76.

Williamson, Ann M., and Anne-Marie Feyer. "Moderate Sleep Deprivation Produces Impairments in Cognitive and Motor Performance Equivalent to Legally Prescribed Levels of Alcohol Intoxication." *Occupational and Environmental Medicine* 57, no. 10 (2000): 649–55.

Wilson, Stephanie J., Lisa M. Jaremka, et al. "Shortened Sleep Fuels Inflammatory Responses to Marital Conflict: Emotion Regulation Matters." *Psychoneuroendocrinology* 79 (2017): 74–83.

Wilson, Timothy D., David A. Reinhard, et al. "Just Think: The Challenges of the Disengaged Mind." *Science* 345, no. 6192 (2014): 75–77.

Withers, Rachel. "8 Women Who Were Warned, Given an Explanation, and Nevertheless, Persisted." *Bust,* https://bust.com/feminism/19060 -kamala-harris-tweets-women-who-persisted.html.

Witvliet, C. V. O., A. J. Hofelich Mohr, et al. "Transforming or Restraining Rumination: The Impact of Compassionate Reappraisal Versus Emotion Suppression on Empathy, Forgiveness, and Affective Psychophysiology." *Journal of Positive Psychology* 10 (2015): 248–61.

Xi, Bo, Dan He, et al. "Short Sleep Duration Predicts Risk of Metabolic Syndrome: A Systematic Review and Meta-Analysis." *Sleep Medicine Reviews* 18, no. 4 (2014): 293–97.

INDEX

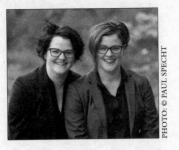

EMILY NAGOSKI is the award-winning author of the *New York Times* bestseller *Come as You Are: The Surprising New Science That Will Transform Your Sex Life*. She has an MS in counseling and a PhD in health behavior, both from Indiana University.

Facebook.com/enagoski
Twitter: @EmilyNagoski

AMELIA NAGOSKI holds a DMA in conducting from the University of Connecticut. An assistant professor and coordinator of music at Western New England University, she regularly presents educational sessions discussing the application of communications science and psychological research for audiences of other professional musicians, including "Beyond Burnout Prevention: Embodied Wellness for Conductors."

## about the type

This book was set in Galliard, a typeface designed in 1978 by Matthew Carter (b. 1937) for the Mergenthaler Linotype Company. Galliard is based on the sixteenth-century typefaces of Robert Granjon (1513–89).